first place

4health

Bible Study Series

start losing
start living

Published by Gospel Light
Ventura, California, U.S.A.
www.gospellight.com
Printed in the U.S.A.

Caution: The information contained in this book is intended to be solely for
informational and educational purposes. It is assumed that the First Place 4 Health
participant will consult a medical or health professional before beginning this or
any other weight-loss or physical fitness program.

Library of Congress Cataloging-in-Publication Data
Start losing, start living.
pages cm. — (First Place 4 Health Bible study series)
ISBN 978-0-8307-6520-1 (trade paper)
1. Christian life—Textbooks. 2. Health—Religious aspects—Christianity—
Textbooks. 3. Joshua (Biblical figure)
BV4511.S727 2013
248.4—dc23
2012044090

Rights for publishing this book outside the U.S.A. or in non-English
languages are administered by Gospel Light Worldwide, an international
not-for-profit ministry. For additional information, please visit
www.glww.org, email info@glww.org, or write to Gospel Light Worldwide,
1957 Eastman Avenue, Ventura, CA 93003, U.S.A.

To order copies of this book and other First Place 4 Health products
in bulk quantities, please contact us at 1-800-727-5223. You can also
order copies from Gospel Light at 1-800-446-7735.

contents

foreword

My introduction to Bible study came when I joined First Place in March 1981. I had been attending church since I was a small child, but the extent of my study of the Bible had been reading my Sunday School quarterly on Saturday night. On Sunday morning, I would listen to my Sunday School teacher as she taught God's Word to me. During the worship service, I would listen to our pastor as he taught God's Word to me. Frankly, the idea of digging out the truths of the Bible for myself had never entered my mind.

Perhaps you are right where I was back in 1981. If so, you are in for a blessing you never dreamed possible. As you start studying the truths of the Bible for yourself through the First Place 4 Health Bible studies, you will see God begin to open your understanding of His Word.

Almost every First Place 4 Health member I have talked with about the program says, "The weight loss is wonderful, but the most important thing I have received from my association with First Place 4 Health is learning to study God's Word." The First Place 4 Health Bible studies are designed to be done on a daily basis. As you work through each day's study (which will take 15 to 20 minutes to complete), you will be discovering the deep truths of God's Word. A part of each week's study will also include a Bible memory verse for the week.

There are many in-depth Bible studies on the market. The First Place 4 Health Bible studies are not designed for the purpose of in-depth study, but are designed to be used in conjunction with the rest of the program to bring balance into your life. Our desire is for each member to begin having a personal quiet time with God each day. This time alone with God should include a time of prayer, Bible reading and Bible study. Having a quiet time is a daily discipline that will bring the rich rewards of balance, which is something we all need.

God bless you as you begin this exciting journey toward a balanced life. God will richly bless your efforts to give Him first place in your life. Remember Matthew 6:33: "But seek first his kingdom and his righteousness, and all these things will be given to you as well."

Carole Lewis, First Place 4 Health National Director

introduction

First Place 4 Health is a Christ-centered health program that emphasizes balance in the physical, mental, emotional and spiritual areas of life. The First Place 4 Health program is meant to be a daily process. As we learn to keep Christ first in our lives, we will find that He is the One who satisfies our hunger and our every need.

This Bible study is designed to be used in conjunction with the First Place 4 Health program but can be beneficial for anyone interested in obtaining a balanced lifestyle. The Bible study has been created in a five-day format, with the last two days reserved for reflection on the material studied. Keep in mind that the ultimate goal of studying the Bible is not only for knowledge but also for application and a changed life. Don't feel anxious if you can't seem to find the *correct* answer. Many times, the Word will speak differently to different people, depending on where they are in their walk with God and the season of life they are experiencing. Be prepared to discuss with your fellow First Place 4 Health members what you learned that week through your study.

There are some additional components included with this study that will be helpful as you pursue the goal of giving Christ first place in every area of your life:

- **Group Prayer Request Form:** This form is at the end of each week's study. You can use this to record any special requests that might be given in class.

- **Leader Discussion Guide:** This discussion guide is provided to help the First Place 4 Health leader guide a group through this Bible study. It includes ideas for facilitating a First Place 4 Health class discussion for each week of the Bible study.

- **Two Weeks of Menu Plans with Recipes:** There are 14 days of meals, and all are interchangeable. Each day totals 1,400 to 1,500 calories and includes snacks. Instructions are given for those who need more calories. An accompanying grocery list includes items needed for each week of meals.

- **First Place 4 Health Member Survey:** Fill this out and bring it to your first meeting. This information will help your leader know your interests and talents.

- **Personal Weight and Measurement Record:** Use this form to keep a record of your weight loss. Record any loss or gain on the chart after the weigh-in at each week's meeting.

- **Weekly Prayer Partner Forms:** Fill out this form before class and place it into a basket during the class meeting. After class, you will draw out a prayer request form, and this will be your prayer partner for the week. Try to call or email the person sometime before the next class meeting to encourage that person.

- **Live It Trackers:** Your Live It Tracker is to be completed at home and turned in to your leader at your weekly First Place 4 Health meeting. The Tracker is designed to help you practice mindfulness and stay accountable with regard to your eating and exercise habits. Step-by-step instructions for how to use the Live It Tracker are provided in the *Member's Guide*.

- **Let's Count Our Miles!** A worthy goal we encourage is for you to complete 100 miles of exercise during your 12 weeks in First Place 4 Health. There are many activities listed on pages 255-256 that count toward your goal of 100 miles. When you complete a mile of activity, mark off the box listed on the Hundred Mile Club chart located on the inside of the back cover.

- **Scripture Memory Cards:** These cards have been designed so you can use them while exercising. It is suggested that you punch a hole in the upper left corner and place the cards on a ring. You may want to take the cards in the car or to work so you can practice each week's Scripture memory verse throughout the day.

- **Scripture Memory CD:** All 10 Scripture memory verses have been put to music at an exercise tempo in the CD at the back of this study. Use this CD when exercising or even when you are just driving in your car. The words of Scripture are often easier to memorize when accompanied by music.

welcome to
Start Losing, Start Living

At your first group meeting for this session of First Place 4 Health, you will meet your fellow members, get an overview of your materials and find out what you can expect at weekly meetings. The majority of your class time will be spent learning about the four-sided person concept, the Live It Food Plan, and how change begins from the inside out. You will also have a chance to ask any questions about how to get the most out of First Place 4 Health. If possible, complete the Member Survey on page 205 before your first group meeting. The information you give will help your leader tailor the next 12 weeks to the needs of the whole group.

Each weekly meeting begins with a weigh-in for members. This will allow you to track your progress over the 12-week session. Your Week One weigh-in/measurement will establish a baseline of comparison so that you can set healthy goals for this session. If you are apprehensive about weighing in every week, talk with your group leader about your concerns. He or she will have some options for you to consider that will make the weigh-in activity encouraging rather than stressful.

The day after your first meeting, begin Week Two of this First Place 4 Health Bible study. During this session, you and your group will un-cover how to step out in faith, draw nearer to God and recognize His power in your life. As you open yourself to the truth of Scripture and share your hopes and struggles with the members of your group during the next 12 weeks, you'll find yourself becoming the healthy child of God you are designed to be!

receive God's blessing

SCRIPTURE MEMORY VERSE
Now the Lord is the Spirit, and where the Spirit of the Lord is, there is freedom.
2 CORINTHIANS 3:17

After 40 years of wandering in the desert, the children of Israel had finally reached the banks of the Jordan River. At long last they were about to enter the Promised Land! However, there appeared to be one final obstacle between God's people and the fulfillment of God's promise: the Jordan River. It was at flood stage, and crossing the raging waters that separated the people from the Promised Land seemed impossible.

Israel's faith, which had been put to the test many times already, was being put to the test once more! However, this time there were no angry Egyptians chasing God's people; there was no urgency pressing them forward. They could have camped by the river until the flood season passed and the waters subsided. After all, God had given territory on the east side of the Jordan to some of the tribes as their inheritance. The other families could have stayed there with them until travel conditions were a bit better. But God, whose timing is always perfect, told them the time to cross the river was *now*:

> After the death of Moses the servant of the LORD, the LORD said to Joshua son of Nun, Moses' aide: "Moses my servant is dead. Now then, you and all these people, get ready to cross the Jordan River into the land I am about to give to them—to the Israelites" (Joshua 1:1-2).

And with that direct command, God also gave Joshua a wonderful promise—a promise that would sustain Joshua and the Israelites in the days and months to come:

> Be strong and courageous. Do not be terrified; do not be discouraged, for the LORD your God will be with you wherever you go (Joshua 1:9).

God is making that same promise to you today as you stand at the threshold of an exciting new adventure into health, wholeness and balanced living. Yes, you could postpone starting this journey for a season or two; however, as it was with the children of Israel, so it is with you. Procrastination is simply not an option! This Bible study is God's voice calling you to swing into action! It is time to *start losing, start living!*

Yes, there are rivers to cross, walls to break down and hurdles to overcome; but you can be strong and courageous because God has promised to never leave or forsake you. A future full of hope is on the horizon. God is with you to bless you. What more do you need?

CALL ON GOD'S PRESENCE AND POWER

Day 1

Sovereign Lord, I am thankful that You are the One leading and guiding me as I begin this exciting adventure. Because You are with me to bless me with Your presence and power, I can stride confidently into a future full of hope. Amen.

Shortly after the Israelites had crossed the Red Sea, they found themselves under attack by hostile enemies. It is at this early point in the exodus that we are introduced to Joshua, whose Battle-of-Jericho fame was yet to come. Please turn in your Bible to Exodus 17:8-16, and read what we first learn about Joshua, who had been born while the Israelites were slaves in Egypt. What did Moses tell Joshua to do (see verse 9)?

Choose some men & fight

While Joshua was occupied, what was Moses going to do (see verse 9)?

Go to the top of the hill and hold the staff up

What did God make happen when Moses raised his arms during Joshua's battle with the Amalekites? What happened when Moses lowered his arms (see verse 11)?

Joshua's Troops were winning when raised losing when lowered

Over time, Moses grew tired. How did Aaron and Hur help (see verse 12)?

They held his arms up

When Moses lifted his hands, what was he really doing (see also Exodus 9:29 and 17:16)?

Lifting his hands to the throne of God

What can you do to be like Moses and invite God's presence and power into your life?

Briefly describe a time when you acted as an Aaron or Hur for someone else or when someone else acted as an Aaron or Hur for you.

_____

_____

_____

_____

Prayer is an important element of your *Start Losing, Start Living* journey. And it is vital for a healthy and thriving relationship with God. Spend part of every day in prayer, asking God to be with you and to bless your efforts as you begin this First Place 4 Health adventure and as you continue your faith journey. Through prayer, you call on God for His presence and power!

> *God of power and might, without You I can do no good thing, but in and through You I can do all that You ask of me. Thank You for being my banner with Your presence and power and for giving me the privilege of prayer. Amen.*

REMEMBER GOD WITH THANKSGIVING
Day 2

> *Gracious God, how thankful I am that You are working all things together for Your glory and my good. I know You have led me to this place, at this time, to accomplish Your plan and purpose for my life. As I move forward, I will put my trust in You. Amen.*

Recalling how God has worked in our lives in times past is an important part of our preparation for the skirmishes we are called to fight today and a reminder of God's encouragement. In the Bible passage we looked at yesterday (Exodus 17:8-16), what did God tell Moses to do in verse 14?

Write down what had happened

_____

_____

_____

Why was preserving the memory of what God had done an important thing to do?

So that others would read it and see what God had done

Read Numbers 15:37-41. What did God want the Israelites to remember, and what were they supposed to do to help them remember (see verses 38-39)?

Remember the Commands of the Lord Wear tassels to remind them

Read 1 Corinthians 11:23-26. At the Last Supper, what did Jesus tell us to do as a way to remember what He did for us (see verses 24-25)?

The Lord's Supper

What symbols or things help you remember an important event or instruction?

Being thankful is all about remembering. Read 1 Chronicles 16:8-12. When he remembered all that God had done for His people, what did David say to do?

Give thanks, sing praises, rejoice

Take a few minutes to think over the events of the past few days. Think back and remember whether you thanked God for everything that happened. Remembering that God is always with you will prompt you to always be thankful!

All-powerful God, thank You for bringing to my mind all that You have done for me and all that You do for me every day. I am truly thankful, though I know that I don't always remember to say so. Help me to remember You first and to always have a grateful heart. Amen.

RELY ON GOD'S PROMISES

Day 3

Thank You, loving Lord, for giving me Your very great and precious promises so that I can share in the abundant life Jesus promised to those who believe in Him. Amen.

Scripture tells us that prior to the time he was anointed to lead the children of Israel into the Promised Land, Joshua believed in God's promises and took God at His word. We need to do the same. Read Numbers 13:26-33. After the spies had explored the Promised Land, what report did the majority of spies give (see verses 27-29)?

_____

_____

_____

_____

_____

What did Caleb say the Israelites should do? How would you describe his attitude (see verse 30)?

_____

_____

_____

_____

How did the other spies respond to the suggestions that Caleb made (see verses 31-33)?

_____

_____

_____

_____

_____

Read Numbers 14:1-9. What did the people think of the leadership of Moses and Aaron (see verses 1-4)?

_____

_____

_____

_____

_____

What did both Joshua and Caleb suggest the people do, and why did they think the action would be possible (see verses 7-9)?

_____

_____

_____

_____

_____

God blesses those who trust in Him. According to the following verses, what are some of the things that God has promised to give those who belong to Him?

John 10:28: _____

John 14:27: _____

Acts 2:38: _____

Philippians 4:13: _____

Read Romans 4:13-16. What was required of Abraham for him to receive the promises of God?

_____

_____

_____

_____

> *Thank You, precious Lord, for revealing Yourself to me in new and exciting ways. Your very great and precious promises give me strength and courage. You are with me to bless me, and I am grateful. Amen.*

PREPARE YOURSELF FOR GOD

Day 4

> *Lord God, as I seek to follow Your precepts, help me to be worthy to receive all that You have prepared for me. Help me to sanctify myself so that I am worthy of Your many blessings. Amen.*

After Moses died, the time had finally come for Joshua to assume the position for which the Lord had been preparing him: Joshua was to lead God's Chosen People into the Promised Land. Turn in your Bible to Joshua 3. What were the people told to do before crossing the Jordan (see verse 5)?

_____

_____

_____

_____

To "consecrate" means to dedicate something or someone for a sacred purpose. For what did God want His people to be prepared (see verse 5)?

_____

_____

_____

_____

What specifically did God do to show the people that He was with them (see verse 13)?

_____

_____

_____

_____

_____

Look up the word "sanctify" in a dictionary. What does the word mean?

_____

_____

_____

_____

According to 1 Thessalonians 5:22-24, how are we sanctified?

_____

_____

_____

_____

Now look at John 17:17. What is the "truth" that sanctifies us?

_____

_____

_____

_____

Read Hebrews 4:12-13. How does God's Word work in us?

_____

_____

_____

_____

What are three specific things you can do so that God's Word works within you?

1. _____

2. _____

3. _____

Dear God, please continue Your work in me so that I may honor You with my being. Thank You for loving me, even though I am sometimes less-than-holy in Your eyes. Amen.

WALK IN FREEDOM   Day 5

Thank You, Lord. Because Your Spirit dwells in me, I can visualize what true freedom looks like. I trust You to have more good things in store for me than I could possibly imagine. Amen.

This week's memory verse describes why every believer walks in true freedom. Write from memory 2 Corinthians 3:17.

_____

_____

_____

What specifically does God give to every person who believes in Jesus (see also 1 Corinthians 2:12)? What does this gift help us do?

_____

_____

_____

_____

According to Romans 8:9, how does the Spirit impact the life of a believer?

_____

_____

According to 2 Corinthians 3:6, what does the Spirit give us?

_____

_____

_____

Paul says that "since we live by the Spirit," we should do what (see Galatians 5:25)? What does this create in our lives (see verses 22-23)?

_____

_____

_____

According to Psalm 119:45, what is the best way for us to continue to walk in freedom?

_____

_____

_____

What does James 1:25 say "the perfect law" gives?

_____

_____

_____

_____

When put into the context of your First Place 4 Health endeavors, what does a walk in freedom look like to you? List three specific ways in which you want to walk in freedom:

1. _____

2. _____

3. _____

How magnificent are Your words to me, O God! Wonder of wonders, You love me with an everlasting love. Your goodness to me knows no bounds. Amen.

REFLECTION AND APPLICATION

Ever-present, ever-loving God, what joy I find in Your presence, what security there is in Your unfailing love! As I learn more and more about You, I am learning to claim Your very great and precious promises as my own. Thank You for loving me. Amen.

"O LORD, how many are my foes! . . . Many are saying of me, 'God will not deliver him'" (Psalm 3:1-2). David penned Psalm 3 at a particularly anxious time in his life, a time when enemies threatened to destroy him. Those "foes" were the hostile armies that posed a threat to David's physical safety and security, but David's enemies were not limited to the hostile people who outwardly opposed him. David's enemies included the people who said to him, "There is no help for you in God."

Indeed, for most of us, the hostile forces that assail us are usually not physical people. Rather, the foes that most often rise up against us are the negative beliefs that repeat themselves over and over again in our heads. And, although the poisonous messages vary depending on our circumstances, the bottom line of every message is the same: "God is not with you to bless you. God won't help you." There is absolutely no outside enemy who can damage our safety and security as quickly as those inner enemies that convince us that God is not with us; that the Lord of heaven's armies will not protect us, deliver us and provide for us.

Reflect for a moment on the negative messages that threaten your safety and security in God. What message (or two or three) bothers you the most?

_____

_____

_____

_____

No matter what those inner hostile voices say, Scripture assures us that God is always with us and that He longs to bless us. And for that we should praise and thank Him always: "Praise be to the God and Father of our Lord Jesus Christ, who has blessed us in the heavenly realms with every spiritual blessing in Christ" (Ephesians 1:3).

We are promised that our Lord will never leave us or forsake us. God "has given us his very great and precious promises" (2 Peter 1:4). He has endowed us with the power of prayer. We have everything we need to succeed as we *start losing, start living.*

Today is the day to allow God's gracious Spirit to fill you with peace and joy as you trust in Him. When you center your mind and heart with the truth of God's Word, there is no room for voices that tell you there is no hope for us in God. You can silence those voices with God's Word!

Today, gracious God, I will go forward toward the good things You have in store for me because You have promised to never leave me or forsake me. Freedom is mine because Your Son has set me free to love and serve You. Amen.

Day 7

REFLECTION AND APPLICATION

Thank You, all-knowing God. Before I face a challenge, You have prepared a solution. As I walk forward in faith, You go with me to bless me. How grateful I am for Your abiding presence and many blessings. How thankful I am that You are always with me wherever I go. Amen.

In a world filled with empty promises, God's Word gives us strength to take on whatever challenges God calls us to face. We can be strong and courageous because our God is with us to bless us! The promises that God made to Joshua—and the Israelites—when the Lord called them to cross over into the Promised Land, God also makes to us:

I will give you every place where you set your foot, as I promised Moses. Your territory will extend from the desert to Lebanon, and from the great river, the Euphrates—all the Hittite country— to the Great Sea on the west. No one will be able to stand up against you all the days of your life. As I was with Moses, so I will be with you; I will never leave you nor forsake you (Joshua 1:3-5).

Think about the first promise: "I will give you every place where you set your foot." What application do those words have as you travel toward balanced living emotionally, spiritually, mentally and physically?

_____

_____

_____

_____

The second promise, "No one will be able to stand up against you," is an assurance that we will defeat our enemies. What enemies do you need to conquer as part of your commitment to the First Place 4 Health program? (Remember that enemies can be attitudes and self-talk as well as people who oppose your goals.)

_____

_____

_____

_____

"As I was with Moses, so I will be with you; I will never leave you nor forsake you" are the third and fourth promises. How will the fact that God is with you and will never leave you help you reach your First Place 4 Health goals?

_____

_____

_____

_____

All-powerful God, I have heard Your voice, and I know that You are calling me to move forward with You on this exciting journey to living a balanced life. I am blessed by having Your Spirit within me, and I am confident that You will continue to bless me as I strive to reach my life goals. Amen.

Group Prayer Requests

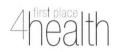

Today's Date: _____

Name	Request

Results

_____

_____

_____

_____

_____

Week Three

step out
in faith

SCRIPTURE MEMORY VERSE
But you are a chosen people, a royal priesthood, a holy nation, a people belonging to God, that you may declare the praises of him who called you out of darkness into his wonderful light.
1 PETER 2:9

As God's people made the necessary preparations for crossing the Jordan River, Joshua sent two spies into the land that God's people would soon inhabit. Unlike the 12 spies Moses had sent into the Promised Land some 40 years earlier, these two men came back with an excellent report and told the Israelite people: "The LORD has surely given the whole land into our hands; all the people are melting in fear because of us" (Joshua 2:24).

Three days later, the officers went through the camp, directing the people: "When you see the ark of the covenant of the LORD your God, and the priests, who are Levites, carrying it, you are to move out from your positions and follow it" (Joshua 3:3).

Joshua ordered the priests to take up the Ark of the Lord and step into the raging Jordan River. Although the people had never been in this place before, the Lord assured them that the Ark of the Covenant (which represented God's presence among them) would show them the way. Through Joshua, the Lord assured the Israelites that just as soon as the priests' feet touched the water's edge, the water flowing downstream would be stopped and pile up (see Joshua 3:13).

And that is exactly what happened! God was indeed with His people to bless them. Just as the children of Israel had crossed the Red Sea on dry land 40 years earlier, God's people walked across the Jordan River on dry ground!

Joshua's story is pertinent to our faith journey because there are many times in our lives when God asks us to step into "raging water" as a sign of obedience and trust. Making a commitment to enter into a deeper relationship with God is one of those times. However, we will never see the amazing things our gracious God can do for us until we are willing to take that first step of faith!

Day
1

FAITHFUL OBEDIENCE

Spirit of love and power, I am so thankful that You are always with me, guiding my steps and showing me the way to live a life pleasing to God. Amen.

As it was with the children of Israel, so it is with us: When God calls us to step forward in faith He always assures us that, even if we don't know how to do this new thing, His Spirit will go with us to show us the way. Read Nehemiah 9:16-21. In this recounting of the story of Moses, how did the people repeatedly react to the commands God had given them (see verses 16-17)?

_____

_____

_____

_____

What did God do in response (see verses 17-18)?

_____

_____

_____

_____

_____

When the Israelites wandered in the desert, what specifically did God give them so that they would know what to do (see verses 19-20)?

_____

_____

_____

_____

_____

How did God provide for them (see verse 21)?

_____

_____

_____

Read John 14:15,21-23. According to Jesus, how do we show we love God?

_____

_____

_____

According to Luke 11:28, what did Jesus say would happen when we obey God's commands?

_____

_____

_____

_____

According to 1 John 2:3-6, what does our obedience show?

_____

_____

_____

The Bible is the obvious source of knowledge about God's commands, but why is it so reliable (see 2 Timothy 3:16-17)?

_____

_____

_____

_____

_____

Thank You, merciful Father, for sending Jesus to show me how to live a life that is pleasing to You. Obedience is the prelude to seeing amazing things. Today I will step forward in faith so that You can bless me. Amen.

Day
2

A ROYAL PRIESTHOOD

Gracious God, You have given me all I need to live a life of godliness through the spiritual blessings that are mine in Christ Jesus my Lord. Help me to be true to the plan and purpose You have for my life. Amen.

Before Jesus Christ came to earth in human form, there was a clear distinction between the common people and those chosen to be priests. Read Hebrews 5:1-4. What were the priests chosen to do?

_____

_____

_____

_____

However, when Jesus Christ became our great High Priest, all that changed. Now look at Hebrews 10:1-14. What could the animal and other such sacrifices never do (see verses 1,3-4,11)?

_____

_____

_____

_____

What did Jesus' sacrifice do so that all previous sacrifices were no longer necessary (see verse 10)?

_____

_____

_____

_____

What does verse 14 tell us about those for whom Jesus made His sacrifice?

_____

_____

_____

_____

Why was the sacrifice Jesus made an acceptable offering to God (see Hebrews 9:12,14)?

_____

_____

_____

_____

This week's memory verse tells us an incredible truth about the priesthood that was ushered in by the new covenant established by Christ Jesus our Lord. Write from memory 1 Peter 2:9.

_____

_____

_____

According to our memory verse, what is our relationship to God, and what does this suggest about how we should live our lives?

_____

_____

_____

_____

How is your participation in First Place 4 Health an opportunity to declare God's praises?

_____

_____

_____

_____

> *Jesus, You are my great High Priest, the perfect sacrifice that has made me right with God. Help me to declare Your praises in all I say and do. Amen.*

Day 3 — TUMBLING STRONGHOLDS

O Lord, You are the one who guides my steps and keeps me safe. Because You are always with me, I am assured of victory over my strongholds. Amen.

As children, many of us learned a song about Joshua and the battle he fought at Jericho. Maybe you at least remember these words from the old spiritual:

> *Joshua fought the battle of Jericho, Jericho, Jericho,*
> *Joshua fought the battle of Jericho,*
> *And the walls came tumblin' down.*

Even though those lyrics may be familiar, you may not remember the details of that mighty feat. Turn in your Bible to Joshua 6:1-21. What did God command Joshua to do in order to defeat Jericho (see verses 3-5)?

_____

_____

_____

According to verses 18-19, what additional instructions did God give?

_____

_____

_____

Because the people followed God's instructions, what did God do to the stronghold of Jericho (see verse 20)?

_____

_____

_____

_____

Although we will probably not need to knock down the physical walls of a city stronghold, we do face "strongholds" on us that can keep us from having a thriving relationship with God. Read 2 Corinthians 10:3-5. What sort of strongholds do we need to destroy (see verse 5)?

_____

_____

_____

_____

What do we use to break down the walls that separate us from God (see verse 4)? What is our goal in destroying these strongholds (see verse 5)?

_____

_____

_____

_____

Now read Ephesians 6:10-18. What are our primary offensive weapons against the devil and his schemes (see verses 17-18)?

_____

_____

_____

_____

Think about the things of this world that might hold you back from a closer relationship with God or from the truth of God's Word. What do you need to get rid of in order to live a balanced life emotionally, spiritually, mentally and physically?

_____

_____

_____

_____

_____

You, O God, are steadfast and strong. You always do what You have promised. Teach me to use the truth of Your Word to demolish the strongholds in my life that keep me from a closer relationship with You. Thank You for Your faithfulness and Your love. Amen.

Day 4 — UNCONFESSED SIN

O Lord, You are always true to Your word, even when Your voice contains a warning I fail to heed. I am thankful that You forgive my sins and choose to remember them no more, for I am a sinner saved only by Your grace. Amen.

The Israelites had an astounding victory at Jericho, but then things went terribly wrong. Read Joshua 7:1-13. What report did the spies give to Joshua about Ai (see verses 2-3)?

_____

_____

_____

_____

_____

What happened when the Israelites went against Ai (see verses 4-5)?

_____

_____

_____

_____

What did Joshua do in response (see verses 6-9)?

_____

_____

_____

_____

Why did things go as they did in Ai (see verses 1,11-12; see also Joshua 6:18-19)?

_____

_____

_____

_____

What had Achan done (see Joshua 7:20-21)?

_____

_____

_____

Achan's sin had severe consequences for the whole nation of Israel and had to be dealt with. Once that was taken care of (read Joshua 7:22-26 for the details), what did God tell Joshua (see Joshua 8:1-2)?

_____

_____

_____

_____

Do you have any "secret sins" that you have not been willing to let go of—sins that keep you from reaping God's rich blessings? If so, ask God to show you any sins that are hidden or that you have forgotten about, and ask for His forgiveness.

Thank You, Lord, that when I confess my sins, You are faithful to forgive me, to remember my sins no more and to help me turn back to You. Amen.

SINCERE CONFESSION

Dear Lord, You are awesome! You do not allow me to wallow in my
sin and wrongdoing; rather, You invite me to confess my sins so that I
can once again be right with You. Amen.

Unconfessed sins keep us from receiving God's blessings and favor. Turn
in your Bible to 1 John 1:8-10. Why is it so important that we acknowledge and confess our sins to God (see verse 8)?

_____

_____

_____

_____

_____

What does God do when we confess our sins (see verse 9)?

_____

_____

_____

_____

What are the consequences for not admitting we have sinned (see verse 10)?

_____

_____

_____

_____

Read Ephesians 2:8-10. By what are we saved, and how can we earn that
(see verses 8-9)?

_____

_____

_____

_____

_____

Once we believe in Jesus, what does God expect us to do (see verse 10)?

_____

_____

_____

_____

_____

Why does God expect us to do those things (see also Ephesians 4:12-13)?

_____

_____

_____

_____

_____

You, O God, are Spirit and You are truth. Thank You for giving me an opportunity to come to You in confession, trusting that You have forgiven my sins through the perfect sacrifice of Your Son. Amen.

REFLECTION AND APPLICATION

Day
6

Over and over again You assure me, loving God, that You not only forgive my sins, but that You also remember them no more. Because of that truth, I can look forward to a future filled with hope. Thank You! Amen.

The second chapter of Joshua tells about an interesting woman named Rahab. Before the Israelites crossed the Jordan River into Canaan, Joshua sent two spies into the Promised Land to scout out the nearby territory in and around Jericho. When the spies were in that city, Rahab sheltered the spies in her home.

When the king of Jericho learned that some spies were in his territory, he sent a message to Rahab that she should turn over the spies to him. Rahab, however, said that though the spies had indeed been at her house, they had left before the gate to the city was shut for the night.

Then she pointed out that if the king's men hurried, they probably could catch up with the spies and capture them. The king's men left in pursuit of the spies, and the city gate closed behind them.

Meanwhile, Rahab, whose life was now in a precarious position, went up to the roof of her house—where she had hidden the spies under some flax that was laid out to dry. Rahab spoke to the spies, suggesting a way for them to return safely to the Israelite camp and at the same time suggesting a way to make sure her own life was saved.

First, Rahab told the spies that she knew that God had given the land to the Israelites, and she told them about the rumors going around about some of the miracles that God had performed for His people: "When we heard of it, our hearts melted and everyone's courage failed because of you, for the LORD your God is God in heaven above and on the earth below" (Joshua 2:11).

Notice that Rahab, a native of Canaan and a worshiper of pagan gods, confesses to the spies that she now has faith in God. (She also tells the spies that the Canaanites are scared of the Israelites, a valuable bit of information for the spies.) Rahab then asks the spies to spare everyone in her family when the Israelites conquer Jericho.

The spies agree, Rahab helps the men escape undetected from the city, and eventually the spies make their way back to Joshua. When the Israelites do conquer Jericho, Rahab and her family are spared (see Joshua 6:22-23).

In spite of her dire circumstances and questionable profession (from Hebrews 11:31 and James 2:25, we learn that Rahab was a prostitute), Rahab was a woman who trusted God. And because of her faith in God, Rahab and her entire family were saved. But the rich rewards of Rahab's faith in God did not end there.

The genealogy at the end of the book of Ruth tells us that Rahab became the mother of Boaz and the great, great grandmother of King David (see Ruth 4:18-22). And if that were not enough, Rahab went on to become one of the five women listed in Matthew's genealogy of Jesus, the Christ (see Matthew 1:1-17)!

As you reflect on this story, what are the benefits of us, like Rahab, placing ourselves under the umbrella of God's protection?

_____

_____

_____

_____

In what ways have your belief and trust in God given you hope for the future?

_____

_____

_____

_____

Gracious God, how wonderful it is to read stories of faith that inspire me to trust in You. Thank You for giving me the example of Rahab, who became part of the great family of God because of her faith in You. Amen.

REFLECTION AND APPLICATION

Day
7

Loving Lord, thank You for Your Word and Your promises and for the men and women of Scripture who inspire me to live a life pleasing to You. Amen.

Often we read about the men and women whose stories are told in the pages of Scripture without giving much thought as to why God chose to include them in the Bible. But God never does anything without having a very good reason for doing so—whether we understand His reasoning or not!

Although God is certainly not obliged to tell us why He does what He does, through the words of the apostle Paul, God tells us exactly why the stories of some people take up space in the Bible: "For everything that was written in the past was written to teach us, so that through endurance and the encouragement of the Scriptures we might have hope" (Romans 15:4).

Everything that was written in the past was written for our benefit. Every person and every story in the Bible has a lesson to teach us. So far in our *Start Losing, Start Living* Bible study, we have learned the stories of some of God's people who have valuable lessons to teach those of us living in the light of God's love today. Write what lesson you learned from reading the stories of the persons listed below, and also include how each story has encouraged you and given you hope.

Joshua

_____

_____

_____

_____

The two spies sent by Joshua into the Promised Land ahead of God's people

_____

_____

_____

_____

Rahab

_____

_____

_____

_____

The priests who carried the Ark of the Covenant into the raging water

_____

_____

_____

_____

As you pray to God today, thank Him for including so many people's stories in His Word so that you might be encouraged in your faith and filled daily with new hope.

You are so very good to me, Lord! Even the stories in the Bible that I am prone to skim over—or ignore altogether—have a valuable lesson to teach me. Help me to learn lessons from those who have gone before me so that my story can become an example of hope and inspiration to others. Amen.

Group Prayer Requests

4 first place
health

Today's Date: _____

Name	Request

Results

_____

_____

_____

_____

_____

win over
deception

SCRIPTURE MEMORY VERSE
And whatever you do, whether in word or deed, do it all in the name of the Lord Jesus, giving thanks to God the Father through him.
COLOSSIANS 3:17

As the story of Joshua and the children of Israel continued to unfold, God fulfilled His promise to drive the hostile people out of the land that the Lord had promised to give His people as their inheritance. Because the people obeyed God and had the courage to step into the raging waters, they were able to claim the Lord's promises and inhabit the land. Soon, with God's help, they began to take possession of all the main areas of Canaan.

However, before Joshua led the people forward, he learned from God that the people needed to reestablish a right position with God and recognize and acknowledge who was in control. Nothing that was being done was happening through their own power. We must recognize and acknowledge the same thing.

Also like the Israelites, we must remember that our God is mightier than any obstacle we face. We "simply" have to remain faithful to God and follow His commands. The same faithful Lord who promised to be with the Israelites and bless them will allow us to begin enjoying the benefits of our efforts in the First Place 4 Health program, even before we have completed all He is asking us to do. God's rich blessing and provision are ours to enjoy, even as we press on toward our goals.

DO WHAT GOD REQUIRES

Almighty and powerful God, You have brought me to this place at this time. Please help me to be faithful to the lessons I am learning through the First Place 4 Health program. I want to discipline myself to live a balanced life that pleases You. Amen.

After they crossed the Jordan River—even before they conquered Jericho and Ai—the Chosen People camped at Gilgal. Read Joshua 5:2-12. What did God require of the Israelites (see verses 2-3)?

_____

_____

_____

_____

Why did God require this (see verses 4-7)?

_____

_____

_____

_____

What else did the people do at Gilgal (see verses 10-12)?

_____

_____

_____

_____

Of what did this celebration remind the Israelites (see Exodus 12, if you don't remember what happened)?

_____

_____

_____

_____

Read Joshua 8:30-35. After the conquest of Jericho and Ai, what did Joshua, along with the entire company of the children of Israel, do?

_____

_____

_____

_____

Why do you think this was necessary?

_____

_____

_____

_____

What should we do daily so that we remember who is in control and so that we'll know what is required of us?

_____

_____

_____

_____

Faithful Father, as I continue this journey with You, I ask for the courage to be disciplined to follow whatever You require of me. Help me to keep You first in all things. Amen.

ASK GOD FIRST

Day 2

Lord God, help me to always consult with You before I make commitments so that I do not do anything that is contrary to Your will and way. Amen.

Throughout salvation history, we see a pattern that repeats itself: Whenever someone makes a commitment to love and serve God at a deeper level, the devil is always lurking in the shadows, ready to transform that commitment into an occasion for failure. Read Joshua 9. When the kings in the region heard about all that God's Chosen People had done to Jericho and Ai, what did the kings do (see verses 1-2)?

_____

_____

_____

What did the people of Gibeon do when they heard what Joshua had done to Jericho and Ai (see verses 3-6)?

_____

_____

_____

What story did the Gibeonites tell Joshua, and what proof did they offer as evidence that they were telling the truth (see verses 9-13)?

_____

_____

_____

What did the men of Israel do—and what did they fail to do—before Joshua made a peace treaty with the people of Gibeon (see verse 14)?

_____

_____

_____

What did the Israelites do when they learned that they had been deceived (see verses 18-21,26-27)?

_____

_____

_____

Think of a time when you chose to take an action without inquiring of the Lord. What was the result? How could/did your action place you in jeopardy with regard to living a healthy, balanced, God-honoring life?

_____

_____

_____

_____

_____

When we began this *Start Losing, Start Living* Bible study, we made a new commitment—or renewed a previous commitment—to live a life that will allow us to achieve our goals to live a balanced life emotionally, spiritually, mentally and physically. What truth do we need to remember lest we, too, fall victim to a ruse?

_____

_____

_____

_____

_____

Gracious God, You are the source of all wisdom. Help me to always inquire of You before I enter into agreements or believe anything that may sabotage my goal of always keeping You first in my life. Amen.

CLAIM GOD'S FAITHFULNESS

Day **3**

Merciful and compassionate Lord, how thankful I am that Your faithfulness remains, even though I sometimes make mistakes and bad decisions. Your love and Your gift of grace mean so very much to me. Amen.

Even though Joshua and the people of Israel had failed to inquire of the Lord before making a treaty with the Gibeonites, God remained faithful to His covenant with His Chosen People. God's love and His promises remained. Turn to Joshua 10:1-14. How did the Gibeonite treaty put Israel at risk (see verses 1-6)?

_____

_____

_____

_____

What did God promise Joshua (see verse 8)?

_____

_____

_____

_____

_____

In what specific ways was God faithful to His word (see verses 10-14)?

_____

_____

_____

_____

What does Lamentations 3:19-24 tell us about God's faithfulness? How does remembering this during difficult times help us?

_____

_____

_____

_____

Now read 1 Corinthians 10:12-14. How else is God faithful?

_____

_____

_____

_____

How can we be sure that God will always be faithful and never forget us (see what God says in Isaiah 49:16)?

How does this truth give you renewed hope and courage to press on toward your goals?

> *Thank You, O gracious Lord, for being faithful to me and keeping every one of Your promises to me. Whenever I doubt You, I will remember that You have my name in the palms of Your hands. Amen.*

LET GOD FIGHT

Day
4

> *Lord of heaven's armies, only in Your might and power will I be able to defeat the enemy forces that keep me from living a life honoring to You. Amen.*

Joshua and his troops did not have to fight their battles alone—and neither do we! According to Deuteronomy 3:21-22, what did Moses tell Joshua before he entered the Promised Land?

Read Exodus 14:13-14. Why did the Israelites have no reason to fear the Egyptians who chased them toward the Red Sea?

_____

_____

_____

_____

The Israelites sang to the Lord after crossing the Red Sea. How did they describe God (see Exodus 15:1-3)?

_____

_____

_____

_____

When Joshua addressed the Israelites for the last time, of what did he remind them (see Joshua 23:1-3)?

_____

_____

_____

_____

Read 2 Chronicles 32:7-8. When the king of Assyria threatened to invade Judah, what reason did Hezekiah give for why the Jews had nothing to fear?

_____

_____

_____

How did the people react to Hezekiah's words (see verse 8)?

_____

_____

_____

_____

How does the psalmist describe God in Psalm 46:1-3?

_____

_____

_____

Why does this description give you confidence that God will fight for you?

_____

_____

_____

God of all creation, thank You for using Your mighty power to
show Your love for me in amazing ways. Teach me that when I need
You to fight for me, all I have to do is ask. Amen.

DO YOUR PART

Day
5

Gracious God, Your Word instructs me to do all things for Your glory.
Help me this day to do all that I am called to do in a manner that
brings honor and praise to You. Amen.

Even as we acknowledge the things God did to help Joshua and the Israelites, we cannot overlook the fact that Joshua and his fighting men
marched into battle. We can never expect the Lord to help us if we are not
willing to do our part. This week's memory verse contains wise advice
on how we are to go about all the things the Lord calls us to do. Write
from memory Colossians 3:17.

_____

_____

_____

According to Ephesians 4:29, what sorts of words are we to avoid?

_____

_____

_____

What should our words do (see also 1 Thessalonians 5:11)?

_____

_____

_____

_____

Look up the following proverbs and tell what each says about what our words can do:

12:18: _____

12:25: _____

15:1: _____

16:21: _____

16:24: _____

Now let's look at what God says about deeds. Read James 2:14-26. How is faith that is not accompanied by right actions described (see verses 17,20,26)?

_____

_____

_____

_____

Although we are saved by God's gift of grace (see Ephesians 2:8-9), what do good works show about our faith?

_____

_____

_____

_____

How thankful I am, Lord, that You do not count my sins against me!
When I look at my words and deeds, I see room for improvement.
Thank You for loving me as I am and for guiding me to be more like You. Amen.

REFLECTION AND APPLICATION

O Lord, thank You for showing me that I cannot worship You on my own terms but must do all things according to Your will. Amen.

Throughout the Bible, we read about God making if-then statements—propositions—that we sometimes misinterpret as being some of God's great and precious promises. Today we are going to learn the difference between promises and propositions so that we won't fall into the trap of confusing the two and possibly end up questioning God's faithfulness because what we thought was a promise did not manifest itself in our lives.

Promises are not predicated on our response. When God makes a promise, He *will* fulfill His word. Nothing can change His eternal decrees. God's promises will always come to pass in God's good time. However, in the case of propositions, another rule applies. When we hear God making an if-then statement, we cannot claim it as a promise without first fulfilling our part of the bargain. As an example, read the proposition found in Deuteronomy 11:22-23:

> If you carefully observe all these commands I am giving you to follow—to love the LORD your God, to walk in all his ways and to hold fast to him—then the LORD will drive out all these nations before you, and you will dispossess nations larger and stronger than you.

We cannot isolate the "then" and claim the promise of God's protection, *until* we have done the work to make the first part of the proposition true by fulfilling our "if" part of the bargain. In other words, we cannot expect God to drive out our enemies until we have carefully observed all the commands He has given us to follow. However, as soon as we do the "if" part, we can be assured that the "then" will also be true. As we do our part, the proposition will become a promise.

Now certainly this is not good news for those who would like benefit without responsibility. But in God's kingdom, if-then is always a proposition; and to claim the benefit, we must first do the work.

To see how if-then propositions work, please complete the following chart. In some verses, both the "if" and the "then" are clearly stated. In other verses, one or both are implied—but the fact that we don't see "if" and "then" does not make the words a promise! As you will see from this exercise, not all the propositions are worded in a positive manner, but you can reword in positive terms those that may appear negative.

Scripture	If	Then
Joshua 24:20		
2 Chronicles 7:14		
Matthew 6:33		
John 15:10		
Romans 10:9		
1 John 1:6		

Now that you have completed the exercise, ask yourself a very logical question: *Am I expecting God to do His part when I have not done mine?*

> *Gracious and loving God, help me to be faithful to the things You call me to do, confident that as I do my part, You will be true to Your word. Amen.*

Day
7

REFLECTION AND APPLICATION

God, forgive me for those times I expect You to bless me, even though I have not held up my end of the bargain. Thank You for correcting me. Amen.

In yesterday's lesson, we learned the difference between propositions and promises and the confusion that results when we mix up the two.

First Place 4 Health is also an if-then proposition. *If* we put God first in all things, *then* we will reap the rewards of a balanced, healthy life. However, we cannot expect to reap the benefits of First Place 4 Health if we have not first done the work!

Having seen examples in Scripture of propositions that require an action on our part before they become promises, today you will create your own if-then chart based on what you learned in this week's study (do what God requires, ask God first, claim God's faithfulness, let God fight, do my part). Your propositions can be stated positively (for example, "If I do what God requires, then God will bless me and help me reach my goals") or negatively (for example, "If I don't do what God requires of me, then God will not favor me and my goals won't be reached"). A sixth blank pair of boxes is provided to create other personal if-then statements.

If	Then

Thank You, Lord, for being my teacher, my mentor and my guide as I learn how to better live a life that is pleasing to You in every aspect: emotionally, spiritually, mentally and physically. Amen.

Group Prayer Requests

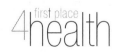

Today's Date: _____

Name	Request

Results

_____

_____

_____

_____

_____

_____

build a legacy of faithfulness

SCRIPTURE MEMORY VERSE
But the fruit of the Spirit is love, joy, peace, patience, kindness, goodness, faithfulness, gentleness and self-control. Against such things there is no law.
GALATIANS 5:22-23

In Joshua 14, we meet a man who has much to teach us about how to build a legacy of faithfulness. Caleb was a man of faith and courage—and a man who understood that his actions were building a legacy for his children and grandchildren in the future:

> Now the men of Judah approached Joshua at Gilgal, and Caleb son of Jephunneh the Kenizzite said to him, "You know what the LORD said to Moses the man of God at Kadesh Barnea about you and me. I was forty years old when Moses the servant of the LORD sent me from Kadesh Barnea to explore the land. And I brought him back a report according to my convictions, but my brothers who went up with me made the hearts of the people melt with fear. I, however, followed the LORD my God whole-heartedly. So on that day Moses swore to me, 'The land on which your feet have walked will be your inheritance and that of your children forever, because you have followed the LORD my God wholeheartedly'" (Joshua 14:6-9).

Caleb was a man who followed his convictions rather than one who was swayed by the opinions of others. When others doubted God's promises, Caleb stood by the Lord, who had promised to always stand by him.

And so it is with us. Future generations will reap untold benefits because of our commitment and faithfulness to God today. What a wonderful gift we can give to our children for generations to come—an inheritance no amount of money could secure.

A SPIRIT OF A DIFFERENT SORT

Heavenly Father, You call me to be faithful in keeping You in the forefront of everything I do. I know that You have good things in store for me. Never let Your gracious hand lose its grip on me. Amen.

Earlier in our Bible study, we learned about Caleb and the courage he and Joshua displayed after he and his companions returned from their spy mission into the Promised Land. Of the 12 spies who went on the mission to spy on the Promised Land, only Joshua and Caleb remembered God's promise to His Chosen People. According to Numbers 14:24, what was the source of Caleb's faithfulness and courage?

_____

_____

_____

_____

Because of Caleb's courage and faith, what two things did God say He would do?

1. _____

2. _____

Read Joshua 14:10-15. What was Caleb's role in God's promise?

_____

_____

_____

_____

What happened as a result (see verse 14)?

_____

_____

_____

Why are some people so easily swayed by the opinions of others?

_____

_____

_____

Look at Romans 12:2. Because believers have the Holy Spirit, a spirit different from what other people have, how should we act in regard to the rest of the world and its opinions?

_____

_____

_____

_____

What should impact and mold our opinions?

_____

_____

_____

_____

According to 1 Thessalonians 5:19-22, what else should we do with what we hear and see?

_____

_____

_____

God, thank You for Your Holy Spirit. Help me to carefully measure the opinions of others and rely on Your Word and promises. I want to live a balanced life that will be part of my legacy to my family and to everyone around me. Amen.

THE REWARDS OF FAITHFULNESS

*Gentle Shepherd, You call for me to be faithful to You, and You promise
that my faithfulness will be rewarded. Thank You for giving me a future
full of hope. Amen.*

Caleb was rewarded by God because he was faithful to serve God with
wholehearted commitment. Look at 1 Samuel 26:23. What does God do
for all those who are faithful to Him?

_____

_____

_____

_____

According to Psalm 37:28, what will God do for those who are faithful
to Him?

_____

_____

_____

_____

According to Proverbs 3:3-4, what will a person win by being faithful
to God?

_____

_____

_____

_____

_____

Now look at Proverbs 16:6-7. How does a man avoid evil?

_____

_____

_____

_____

Even though we may have to go through times of trouble and have to deal with a variety of problems, what will God ultimately give us as a reward if we are faithful to Him (see Revelation 2:10)?

_____

_____

_____

_____

How is steadfast commitment—faithfulness, exercised over time—an essential part of your First Place 4 Health goals?

_____

_____

_____

_____

Dear God, I want to reap all of the rewards You offer to those who are faithful to You alone. Help me have the courage and faith of Caleb. And forgive me for those times I may falter in my commitment to You. Amen.

THE EDUCATION OF FUTURE GENERATIONS

Day 3

You, O Lord, are the God who is the same yesterday, today and forever. Show me how to teach Your ways to future generations. Amen.

The lessons found in the Bible are exactly that: lessons to be learned, applied to our current-day situations and then passed on to future generations. When Moses was reviewing the history of God's people and all that God had done for them and given to them, what did he say was extremely important (see Deuteronomy 4:9)?

_____

_____

_____

_____

According to Deuteronomy 4:40, why was this so important?

_____

_____

_____

_____

According to Deuteronomy 6:6-7, when should children be taught about God and His commands?

_____

_____

_____

_____

Look at Psalm 71:17-18. What does the psalmist ask of God?

_____

_____

_____

_____

What is the benefit of teaching someone when he or she is very young (see Proverbs 22:6)?

_____

_____

_____

_____

According to Ephesians 6:4, how should fathers (and mothers) bring up their children, and what should be avoided (see also Colossians 3:21)?

_____

_____

_____

_____

_____

In what ways does striving to accomplish your First Place 4 Health goals educate members of the younger generation (those in your family, those who see you in church, those who see you as you live out your life in public)?

_____

_____

_____

_____

_____

Thank You, Lord, for allowing me to live my life as a testimony to Your love and faithfulness. Help me to pass on a rich legacy to my descendants and to all future generations. Amen.

SEEDS OF HOPE

Day 4

Gracious God, You offer me so much and ask only for my love. Help me to water the seeds of hope that You have planted in my life so that I flourish in Your light. Amen.

Just as God planted a hope for future blessing in Caleb, so too God gives every believer hope. From where does all hope come (see Psalm 62:5)?

_____

_____

_____

_____

_____

When you are having problems of one sort or another and feeling downcast, what should you do (see Psalm 42:5)?

_____

_____

_____

_____

Read Psalm 130. Even though we might sin, what will God do when we pray to Him (see verses 1-2)?

_____

_____

_____

_____

What does our God offer us when we turn to Him (see verses 3-4)?

_____

_____

_____

_____

Why should we put our hope in God (see verses 7-8)?

_____

_____

_____

_____

When we hope in God, what will He do in our lives (see Isaiah 40:31)?

_____

_____

_____

_____

According to 1 Timothy 6:17, why is hope in God better than any "hope" the world offers?

_____

_____

_____

_____

Read what Paul wants for believers in Christ in Romans 15:13. What are a couple of specific things you can do so that you "overflow with hope"?

_____

_____

_____

_____

Spirit of love and power, when You came to live in my heart You came bearing seeds of hope. Help me to use all You have given me to the glory of God and the benefit of His kingdom so that my hope overflows onto all those around me as they also come to believe. Amen.

AN ABUNDANCE OF FRUIT

Day 5

Dear God, You have given me Your Holy Spirit so that I can produce fruit in my life that will last for generations to come. How fortunate I am to have Your Spirit living in me, telling me that I am a child of God. Amen.

Our memory verse this week tells us that the life lived according to God's Spirit, our source of hope, will produce fruit that will impact everyone we encounter. Write Galatians 5:22-23 from memory.

_____

_____

_____

_____

There are nine fruit of the Spirit, or virtues of Christian character, listed in these two verses from Galatians. Read the Scriptures listed below and tell what other characteristics we should display when we follow Jesus:

Ephesians 4:2: _____

Ephesians 5:8-9: _____

Colossians 3:12-15: _____

Now read Galatians 5:24-26. Because we belong to Christ, what should we do with our sinful nature (see verse 24)?

_____

_____

_____

_____

Also because we belong to Christ, how should we live (see verse 25)?

_____

_____

_____

_____

What should we avoid (see verse 26)?

_____

_____

_____

_____

The fruit of the Spirit is the inheritance of all who believe in Jesus—we were given all those things in equal measures when the Spirit was given to us—but each believer may need to spend more time cultivating and developing one (or more!) of the fruit. Which of the fruit needs your extra attention, and what are a few specific ways you can foster its growth?

_____

_____

_____

_____

Gracious God, You have given me everything I need to live a life of faithfulness and at the same time show Your love to the world through the words I choose to use and the way I choose to live my life. Thank You for empowering me to be all You have created and called me to be in Your Kingdom. Amen.

REFLECTION AND APPLICATION

Almighty and all-powerful God, You work in my life in mysterious ways. You have given me the many fruit of the Spirit so that I can live a life pleasing to You. Help me to be a faithful and fruitful servant who brings joy to my Master. Amen.

During a recent gathering of a Women's Association meeting at church, one of the ladies in the group was describing to the others how she was redecorating her kitchen. She had replaced the floor with imported tile, purchased all new appliances, gotten new window coverings, and painted and papered the walls. Then, in keeping with her new décor, she had hired an artist to paint the "fruit of the Spirit," as described in Galatians 5:22-23, around the ceiling board in vibrant colors that coordinated with the bright new kitchen design and color scheme. She then laughed and said, "All the fruit, that is, except self-control. Self-control isn't something we practice in our kitchen!"

This story may be funny, but not practicing self-control is certainly not a laughing matter. Self-control is remembering what is important and taking the action necessary in order to reach whatever goals and dreams are desired. Without self-control, goals and aspirations are nothing more than wishful thinking. And although we normally think of exercising self-control in regard to food and drink, self-control actually goes beyond the kitchen and whatever eating habits we may be striving to change.

The First Place 4 Health program aims for you to put into practice a lifestyle balanced in every way—emotionally, spiritually, mentally and physically. In order to wholeheartedly commit ourselves to the program, we must earnestly desire, and then claim, the God-given promise of self-control. Self-control is the virtue that allows us to grow and produce fruit that will grace every room in our homes. Without self-control, a person leaves himself or herself open to attacks by the devil (see Proverbs 25:28). When a person practices self-control in every aspect of life, that person has a defensive wall of protection around himself or herself.

Think about the different aspects of a balanced lifestyle and evaluate how you exhibit and/or need to improve self-control in each of them. (For example, do you exercise control of your anger, or are you likely to fly off the handle? Do you worship God faithfully with others or only if your favorite team's game isn't on? Do you let others have their say, or must you always be right? When you're in a social situation, do you eat something you know you shouldn't since everyone else is eating, or do you say "No, thank you"?) Write how you are doing in each area below.

Emotionally

_____

_____

_____

_____

Spiritually

_____

_____

_____

_____

Mentally

_____

_____

_____

Physically

_____

_____

_____

_____

Trust that as you are faithful, God will give more than you can ask for or imagine—both now and throughout eternity.

> *Lord God, You have blessed me with a Spirit of power, of love and of self-discipline. Impress on my heart and mind, in new ways, the importance of being self-controlled in all I do. I want every aspect of the way that I live my life to bring You glory. Amen.*

REFLECTION AND APPLICATION

Day 7

> *Faithful Father, You have promised that as long as the earth endures there will be a sunrise and a sunset and there will be seasons to govern every activity under heaven. Help me to recognize the rhythm of the seasons in my life and to humbly accept my current season of life as a gift from You. Amen.*

The writer of Ecclesiastes tells us that "there is a time for everything, and a season for every activity under heaven" (Ecclesiastes 3:1). In sharp contrast to that is the hurry-up, I-want-it-now, and profit-driven way we live. One of the unfortunate by-products of our haste is that we have lost the wisdom of seasons and the purpose of processes; we have set aside God's concept of "a season for every activity under heaven."

In our obsession with the proverbial bottom line, we have forgotten the essential rhythms created by sowing and reaping, laughing and weeping, sunrise and sunset, rest and work. And in those rhythms, seasons play an essential role. Through it all is God's amazing gift of grace to us, to which we should respond with thankfulness. Too often we fail to see the truth that is before us because we don't take the time to stop and see things from the perspective of Jesus.

We also must understand that all growth—especially spiritual growth—involves seasons. If we fail to recognize that fact, we will become frustrated and wonder why our progress seems so slow at times. In our haste to move forward quickly, we fail to realize that each new spiritual truth we learn must be fed and cultivated, that we must wait for the newly sewn seed to germinate and bear fruit. Even our prayer lives are subject to seasons. As we mature in our faith, we learn to anticipate God's spiritual seasons and not grow weary or lose heart when life seems barren and dark. With time, we realize that winter always precedes the new birth of spring in a world governed by seasons.

Through participation in First Place 4 Health, we come to know that learning to care for ourselves is a process that involves seasons too. There are times when everything is fresh and new, and we see rapid growth. Our burdens become lighter, and our energy levels are high. Sometimes our spiritual seasons correspond with the actual physical seasons. Some of us suffer from lethargy and depression during dark, dreary, wintery weather. Others of us find that we wilt in the humid summer weather, and our bodies prefer the cool, crisp days of fall. Part of the balance of disciplined living is learning to be patient with God and ourselves when our progress is slow and our spiritual growth appears to be dormant.

No matter what season or cycle you are in, there is no reason to grow weary or lose heart. Remember that dark, gloomy days don't last forever; spring always follows winter. Recognize that the rhythms of life apply to everyone. Today is the day to faithfully take the next right step, confident that God's grace will help you develop fruit that will last, because you are living in harmony with God's rhythm of the seasons.

What about God's rhythm of the seasons do you need to more firmly embrace and make your own, and how will that help you accomplish your First Place 4 Health goals?

What have you done to play out the rhythm of the seasons—to show God that you are thankful for His gifts?

_____

_____

_____

_____

_____

_____

Loving Lord, Your grace is incredible. Your great love for me never falters, even when I lose my perspective and take my eye off Jesus and Your kingdom. Thank You for all the gifts You have given to me. Help me to be more active in the rhythm of Your seasons. And help me to walk in harmony with the way You are working in my life. Amen.

Group Prayer Requests

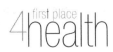

Today's Date: _____

Name	Request

Results

_____

_____

_____

_____

_____

_____

draw nearer to God

SCRIPTURE MEMORY VERSE
Submit yourselves, then, to God. Resist the devil, and he will flee from you.
JAMES 4:7

The book of Deuteronomy, which means "second law," or "repetition of the law," contains Moses' final instructions to God's Chosen People before they entered the Promised Land. The people who listened to Moses' words had been born during Israel's 40 years in the desert. All of those in the original exodus—except Joshua and Caleb—had perished in the desert as a result of their failure to trust God and take Him at His word. Since this was a new generation to whom he was speaking, Moses knew that it was important that he teach them about what God had done for Israel. They needed to know how God had miraculously delivered the Israelites from the cruel bondage of Egypt. Even though the people had grumbled, complained and continually questioned God's presence and God's love, the Lord had been faithful to His covenant promises.

The instructions Moses gave the men and women who would soon enter the Promised Land summarized the essence of Israel's covenant responsibility to God. Moses told the people that the only way they would continue to enjoy God's favor and blessing was through their unswerving love and devotion to the Lord. This was actually a call to action. God's love in action delivered the Jews from Egypt. Israel's love for God was also to be active—and to be demonstrated through their obedience to God's commandments.

As you read Moses' final words to the people, listen to them as if you were standing in the crowd that day, for these words are also words of life for you:

> This day I call heaven and earth as witnesses against you that I have set before you life and death, blessings and curses. Now choose life, so that you and your children may live and that you may love the LORD your God, listen to his voice, and hold fast to him. For the LORD is your life, and he will give you many years in the land he swore to give to your fathers, Abraham, Isaac and Jacob (Deuteronomy 30:19-20).

Choosing to wholeheartedly love and serve God is the most important choice any of us will ever make. We can draw nearer to God and have a blessed and favored life centered in God's promises, or we can choose to have a friendship with the world that brings us nothing that lasts—but we cannot have both. Moses' voice thunders throughout salvation history: "Choose life!"

Day 1

SUBMIT TO GOD

Mighty and powerful Lord, You continually invite me to submit to the plans You have for me. And You give me instructions that ensure me of Your favor and blessing. Thank You for being faithful and true. Amen.

This week's memory verse contains valuable advice for those who have chosen life. Write from memory the words of James 4:7.

_____

_____

_____

_____

_____

_____

When we read James's words, the word "then"—that one seemingly insignificant four-letter word—is actually an invitation to take a look at the context of our memory verse to see why we are being asked to take that action. Read James 4:4-10. What is it that puts us at odds with God (see verse 4)?

_____

_____

_____

_____

_____

What is God's purpose in giving us more grace (see verses 5-6)?

_____

_____

_____

_____

What five things can we do to draw nearer to God (see verses 7-10)?

1. _____

2. _____

3. _____

4. _____

5. _____

What will God do when we do these things (see verse 10)?

_____

_____

_____

_____

Look at Matthew 6:24. What are some of the things people do to show that the world is their master rather than God?

_____

_____

_____

_____

_____

What are a couple of specific practical things you can do in order to resist the devil and show the world that God is whom you serve?

_____

_____

_____

_____

_____

Thank You, loving and merciful God, for giving me Your Word to show me the ways in which I can resist the wiles of the evil one. Today, I humbly submit myself to Your care and teaching. Lord, please help me to continue to draw closer to You. Amen.

Day 2

TAKE ONE STEP AT A TIME

Lord, You know how impatient I am. I would like to have it all—and have it all now! But, in Your wisdom, You outline a step-by-step plan for my growth through Your infinite grace and knowledge. Thank You for being my wise and patient teacher. Amen.

Imagine for a moment that you were among the people as they listened to Moses prepare them to enter the Promised Land. Two emotions undoubtedly prevailed in the minds and hearts of the Israelites as Moses spoke: anticipation and anxiety. Turn in your Bible to Deuteronomy

7:17-26. What reason did Moses give for why the people should not be afraid of the nations they would be facing (see verses 18-21)?

_____

_____

_____

_____

_____

The nations that inhabited the land God had promised to the Israelites did not honor Him and served evil through their idol worship. In order to protect the Israelites, God instructed them to eliminate these nations from the land. Although it would take time for the landscape of Israel to be changed, what did God guarantee would happen (see verses 22-24)?

_____

_____

_____

_____

_____

What were the Israelites to do with the things that did not honor God (see verses 25-26)?

_____

_____

_____

_____

_____

Why was that such an important thing to do (see verse 25)?

_____

_____

_____

_____

Why do you think that just as God helped the Israelites "little by little," He helps us make changes to our lives "little by little" (see verse 22)?

_____

_____

_____

_____

_____

With that in mind, why should we not compare our progress in First Place 4 Health with the progress of others in our group?

_____

_____

_____

_____

_____

Lord, You are my good Shepherd. You know exactly what I need.
You lead and guide me in right paths. You guide and direct my progress,
one step at a time, lifting me higher as I meet each challenge and learn
each lesson before me. Thank You! Amen.

Day 3

CONTINUE TO GROW AS A CHRISTIAN

Thank You, loving Lord, for transforming me into the image of Your
Son, my Savior. As I trust You, You fill me with joy and peace. Amen.

Every life lesson builds on what has come before. Read 2 Peter 1:5-11. How do these verses tell you to build on your faith? What result are you seeking as you grow (see verse 8)?

_____

_____

_____

_____

Why should every believer always work hard to improve his or her relationship with Jesus (see verse 9)?

_____

_____

_____

_____

If we do the things that Peter has suggested, what will happen (see verses 10-11)?

_____

_____

_____

_____

What are some of the specific steps a believer should take in order to "make every effort" to grow as a Christian?

_____

_____

_____

_____

Read Philippians 3:12-14. Why did the apostle Paul "press on," or intentionally seek to serve God and grow in faith?

_____

_____

_____

_____

How would you describe Paul's focus as he pursued God (see verse 13)?

_____

_____

_____

_____

Do you need to leave anything from your past behind so that you can more easily move forward to accomplish your goals and grow in your faith? If so, what do you need to leave behind?

_____

_____

_____

_____

_____

> *You forgive me, Lord, and invite me to put my sins behind me so that I can walk into a future full of hope. Thank You for being my merciful, compassionate God. Amen.*

Day 4 — PUT ON A NEW SELF

My Lord and my God, You have called me to put off my old self so that I can put on the new life that is mine in Christ Jesus, my Lord. Help me to shed my old ways so that I grow ever closer to You. Amen.

Other people should be able to see a change in us when we become believers. Turn to the apostle Paul's words in Ephesians 4:22-32. What are we to do in regard to the way we used to live, and why (see verses 22-24)?

_____

_____

_____

_____

What specifically are we told to stop doing (see verses 25-31)?

_____

_____

_____

_____

_____

What are we to remove from our lives (see verse 31)?

_____

_____

_____

_____

If we do not put on a new self and these things remain in our lives, what will happen (see verse 30)?

_____

_____

_____

According to verse 32, what are we to do, and why?

_____

_____

_____

Look at Galatians 5:16-21. What are some other characteristics of our old selves (see verses 19-21)?

_____

_____

_____

When we each put on a new self, who helps us to live in a more godly way (see verses 16-18)?

_____

_____

_____

_____

What are some specific ways you can put off the old self and replace it with the new?

_____

_____

_____

_____

_____

Gracious God, help me to understand the value of godly living. I certainly do not want to grieve the Holy Spirit, who dwells within me. Please show me whatever I need to get rid of in my life so that I walk down the right path to draw nearer to You. Amen.

Day 5

TAKE UP YOUR CROSS

Loving Lord, You call me to resist the devil by submitting to You. This too is a process that I undertake one step at a time. Help me be faithful in little as a prelude to receiving more. Amen.

Love for the things of the world can be a barrier that keeps us from experiencing the love the Father desires to lavish on us, His children. Read Mark 8:31-38. When Jesus predicted His own death, what did Peter do (see verse 32)?

_____

_____

_____

_____

What was Jesus' reaction, and why (see verse 33)?

_____

_____

_____

_____

What did Jesus mean when He said that each of His followers must "deny himself" (verse 34)?

_____

_____

_____

_____

_____

_____

In what respect does a follower of Christ "lose" his or her life (verse 35)?

_____

_____

_____

_____

_____

What do nonbelievers spend their lives doing, and what do they gain (see verse 36)?

_____

_____

_____

_____

_____

When people live for this world, what are they in danger of losing (see verse 36)?

_____

_____

_____

_____

_____

_____

Although it is unlikely that any of us will ever be required to literally "take up [our] cross," what should we be willing to do for our faith in Jesus (see verse 34)?

_____

_____

_____

_____

_____

Dear God, teach me to take up my cross daily and to focus on what You desire and have for me. Help me to see that what You have in store for me is so very much better than anything the world has to offer. Amen.

Day 6 REFLECTION AND APPLICATION

Lord, I want to draw nearer to You, and I know that can only happen when I am willing to relinquish the things that keep me from loving You with all my heart, soul, mind and strength. Help me to identify and eliminate those things, replacing them with good things, so that I can enjoy unbroken fellowship with You. Amen.

As Christians, we talk a lot about overcoming the sin patterns that keep us enslaved and separated from God. We recognize that those destructive behaviors keep us from living lives characterized by joy and peace.

However, in our struggle against the forces of evil, all too often we forget that simply eliminating sin is not the goal of the Christian life. We are called to submit *and* resist. To concentrate all of our efforts on overcoming sin is to fall short of our calling in Christ Jesus. As Christ followers, we are to practice the principle of replacement. We are to eliminate sin *and* replace it with righteousness; eliminate the bad and replace it with the good.

The apostle Paul told the believers in Rome that they had been set free from sin, not so that they could do whatever they chose, but so that they could voluntarily become slaves to righteousness (see Romans 6:18). Jesus Christ came to break the chains of sin so that we could choose to replace them with things that please God. Our Lord and Savior redeemed us from a life of slavery to sin so that we could willingly serve Him.

That's why Scripture reading, Scripture memorization and prayer are important parts of our daily regimen in First Place 4 Health. We are striving to break our bondage to the desires of this world and the things that the world deems important—status, wealth, the accumulation of bigger and better things, physical perfection. As we deliberately take in more of God, those worldly bonds are broken. We pull weeds and plant flowers; we eliminate clutter and make room for new life; we replace disordered lives with the spiritual discipline that pleases God. As we replace sin with righteousness and continue to grow in our faith, we replace the bad with the good, the good with the better, and the better with the best.

List three specific ways that you will put the principle of replacement into practice today:

1. _____

2. _____

3. _____

Now put those ways into action!

> Dear God, You have called me to be a slave—a willing servant—
> to only You. Thank You, gracious Lord, for encouraging me to put
> my past behind me. I know that You want only what is best for me,
> and that best is not based in this world. Please hold me up whenever
> I falter and allow a weed to grow in my life. I want my life to be
> a garden filled with only good, godly things. Amen.

REFLECTION AND APPLICATION

*Creator of heaven and earth, let me never forget that You created me
in Your image and that You found all You created to be good. I want
my life to bring You glory. Amen.*

We are God's creation! And what did God think of all He created? It was
good! And do you remember in whose image we were created? God's image, of course! After God went to the trouble of creating us, do you really
think that He would abandon something that He had already said was
good? Of course not! This whole idea about being made in God's image
should make it clear that we are not free to simply do what we want with
what God has given us. We are to do all of the things we have been studying this week so that we draw closer and closer to God.

Along with being created in God's image, we also "are the temple of
the living God" (2 Corinthians 6:16). Each of us is God's holy place! The
apostle Paul also wrote: "Do you not know that your body is a temple of
the Holy Spirit, who is in you, whom you have received from God? You
are not your own; you were bought at a price. Therefore honor God with
your body" (1 Corinthians 6:19-20). Because God owns our bodies, we
should not ignore God's standards for living. But because God's Holy
Spirit dwells in us, He is always available to help us do what is right.

We must always be aware that when we do things that do not pro-
mote a balanced lifestyle, we chip away at God's temple. God is not
pleased with us when we do things that contribute to the destruction of
our bodies—or when we fail to do the things that will bring restoration,
balance and healing.

Most of us would prefer not to hear that we are God's holy place, let
alone think about how we've mistreated His temple. But we must consider
what we are doing and not doing in regard to God's temple. Obviously,
participating in this First Place 4 Health Bible study and being an active
participant in the First Place 4 Health program are huge steps in the right
direction. But we must remember that changing to become more like Jesus is a long process that continues as long as we live here on earth.

Take a few moments and think about how you treat God's holy place. Then spend the rest of your quiet time today thinking about the action—or lack of action—that might cause your Creator to wonder about the state of His temple. As you do so, remember that God invites us to confess our sins and shortcomings, not so that He can berate and scold us, but so that He can forgive us and bless us! God loves us too much to allow us to continue in our states of sin!

All-knowing God, You love me just as I am—faults and all. As I walk hand in hand, step by step with You, I will be transformed into the person You created and redeemed me to be in Christ Jesus. Keep before me the fact that Your Holy Spirit dwells in me so that I will be more mindful that I am Yours. I need Your Spirit to guide me as I draw nearer and nearer to You. Amen.

Group Prayer Requests

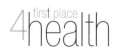

Today's Date: _____

Name	Request

Results

_____

_____

_____

_____

_____

_____

do your part in the race

SCRIPTURE MEMORY VERSE

*Therefore, since we are surrounded by such a great cloud of witnesses,
let us throw off everything that hinders and the sin that so easily entangles,
and let us run with perseverance the race marked out for us.*

HEBREWS 12:1

As the Israelites conquered the land little by little, the descendants of Joseph complained to Joshua because they had only received one allotment and one portion for their inheritance. Genesis 41:50-52 tells us that Joseph had two sons: Manasseh and Ephraim. Technically, it was their father, Joseph, along with Jacob's other eleven sons, who was promised an allotment in the Promised Land. However, just before Jacob died, the aged patriarch promised Joseph that Manasseh and Ephraim would be counted as his own sons with regard to the division of the land God was giving the Israelites (see Genesis 48:3-6).

Because of Jacob's promise to Joseph—and because the descendants of Manasseh and Ephraim were so numerous—Joshua agreed to give them the forest land that adjoined the portion of land they had already received. But, upon hearing Joshua's words, the people of Joseph complained because all of the land had not yet been cleared for settlements and farming. But their complaint did not dissuade Joshua, who insisted that land would be theirs:

> You are numerous and very powerful. You will have not only one allotment but the forested hill country as well. Clear it, and its

farthest limits will be yours; though the Canaanites have iron chariots and though they are strong, you can drive them out (Joshua 17:17-18).

Through Joshua, God was telling Joseph's people they could have the extra portion they deserved; however, they were going to have to work to change the landscape to fit their needs before they could make much use of it. They would have to clear the forest. Today God tells us the same thing about our promised inheritance: If we hope to realize our First Place 4 Health goals, we must be willing to work for them; we must do our part to reach the goals we have.

Day 1 — ELIMINATE ENTANGLEMENTS

God, I want to win the race You have set before me. Help me to eliminate those things that hamper my progress to reach the prize that awaits me. Amen.

In our memory verse this week, the writer of Hebrews uses athletic imagery to make his point. Write from memory Hebrews 12:1.

_____

_____

_____

What does an audience at an athletic event do for the event participants?

_____

_____

_____

Who are some of the people who are watching the race each of us is running (see Hebrews 11)?

_____

_____

_____

How are the witnesses to our race different from the witnesses of a regular athletic event?

_____

_____

_____

Who has designed the course we are racing? What is the goal?

_____

_____

_____

How does sin make running the race difficult?

_____

_____

_____

What is perseverance, and why do we need it to run the race?

_____

_____

_____

Father, help me to realize that I am never alone in my race toward the goal. Other runners before me ran the race and reached the goal. Thank You for telling me about them so I am encouraged and inspired to keep running. Amen.

PRACTICE SELF-DISCIPLINE

Day 2

Dear God, I know that I'm not always the best athlete in the race and that I sometimes fall behind in my "training and conditioning." Thank You for never giving up on me and for loving me as I run. Amen.

Regular athletes condition their bodies so that they are able to run the fastest, leap the highest or in some other way exhibit greater physical stamina and agility than the other athletes in the competition. The apostle Paul tells us how this type of physical excellence is achieved. Read 1 Corinthians 9:24-27. How are we supposed to run (see verse 24)?

_____

_____

_____

_____

In what two ways is the prize we seek different from the prize given to a regular runner (see verses 24-25)?

1. _____

2. _____

In what way are we to be like regular runners (see verse 25)?

_____

_____

_____

_____

What did Paul do that we should also do in regard to training for the race (see verse 27)?

_____

_____

_____

_____

What are some of the things that indicate that a person is "running aimlessly" or "beating the air" (verse 26)?

_____

_____

_____

_____

Read Galatians 5:7-8. What happened to some people whom Paul said had been "running a good race"?

_____

_____

_____

How can other people "cut in" and cause you to stumble as you race toward the prize God has planned for you?

_____

_____

_____

How can other people cut in and cause you to stumble as you race toward your First Place 4 Health goals?

_____

_____

_____

_____

Thank You, gracious Lord, for keeping my eyes on the prize You have set before me. As I am faithful in my practice of self-discipline, help me to avoid people and situations that cut in and try to ruin my race. Amen.

KEEP JESUS IN SIGHT

Day 3

Lord God, there are so many distractions that keep me from doing the good things You call me to do. Only with Your help can I achieve the goal You have set before me. Help me keep my focus where it belongs. Amen.

Let's look at the context of this week's memory verse. Read Hebrews 12:2-3. As we run, on whom should our focus be? Why should He be our focus?

_____

_____

_____

What led Christ to run His race in spite of what He had to endure (see 2 Corinthians 5:21)?

_____

_____

_____

_____

_____

Why should we "not grow weary and lose heart" (verse 3)?

_____

_____

_____

What might happen to a runner who becomes distracted, tired or discouraged?

_____

_____

_____

_____

What are some of the things that can distract us from the One on whom we should focus?

_____

_____

_____

_____

Thank You, Jesus, for always focusing on the prize that awaited You. Help me to be like You and to focus on You so that I too will win the prize. Do not let anything of this world distract me or discourage me. Amen.

HAVE RESPECT FOR YOURSELF

*Creator God, You fashioned and made me in accordance with Your plan and
purpose for my life. You respect all of Your creation, and that includes me.
Guide me to do the same. Amen.*

We need to have the same respect for what God created that He has for
all He created. And that includes ourselves—our bodies. Read Psalm
139:1-18. What does God know about us (see verses 1-4)?

_____

_____

_____

_____

Where is God as each person lives his or her life (see verses 5,18)?

_____

_____

_____

Why can we never be lost to God (see verses 7-10)?

_____

_____

_____

How were each of us created? Why should this lead us to praise God (see
verses 13-16)?

_____

_____

_____

How often does God think of us (see verses 17-18)?

_____

_____

_____

Does knowing that God's Spirit is always with you cause you comfort or fear, and why?

_____

_____

_____

How does knowing that God is always with you affect the way you think and behave?

_____

_____

_____

Dear God, I know that I am a miracle created by You. Keep me mindful that You are always with me and that You truly love and accept me as I am. Help me to show myself the same respect, love and acceptance. Amen.

Day 5

STOP MAKING EXCUSES

You, O God, call me to be accountable for all I say and do. Help me to remember that fact. I know that there really is no justification for not doing what I should to live a balanced life. Amen.

People have been making excuses for their poor behavior for a very, *very* long time. Read Genesis 3:8-13. What were Adam and Eve's excuses for eating the forbidden fruit (see verses 12-13)?

_____

_____

_____

Now look at Luke 14:16-24, the parable of the great banquet. What were the excuses given for not attending the banquet (see verses 18-20)?

_____

_____

_____

How did the host respond to the excuses (see verses 21-23)?

_____

_____

_____

_____

What did the host say would happen to the original invited guests (see verse 24)?

_____

_____

_____

Read James 1:13-15. Who is ultimately responsible for wrong thoughts and actions (see verse 14)?

_____

_____

_____

_____

Now look at Exodus 4:10-12. When Moses kept giving God excuses for not wanting to be the one to confront Pharaoh, what did God point out to him (see verse 11)?

_____

_____

_____

_____

What are some of the excuses you've heard people use for not doing what was right?

_____

_____

_____

_____

How do excuses hinder us from running the race that God has called us to win?

_____

_____

_____

_____

Dear God, thank You for not letting me get away with any excuses I try to use to justify my wrong thoughts and actions. Teach me that I can do all things, because You are always with me, and You strengthen me. I know that nothing is too difficult for You. Amen.

Day 6

REFLECTION AND APPLICATION

O Lord God, You have given me everything I need to live a life pleasing to You, which includes pointing out that I need to do my part in the race You have set before me. Thank You for meeting all my needs. Amen.

If you are like most people, you've occasionally felt as though you have too much to do and not enough time to get it all done! Perhaps that is so because of how easy it is to think purely in terms of material things when we consider God's promise of provision (see Philippians 4:19).

However, God has promised to give us *everything* we need—and everything includes having enough time and energy to do the things God calls us to do. For most of us, time is our most valuable resource, mainly because we all get a 24-hour-per-day time allotment—no more, no less. If we use up today's ration, we have to wait until tomorrow to get a new supply. When it comes to managing ourselves in relation to time, the apostle Paul gives us solid advice in Ephesians 5:15-17. What does Paul tell us?

_____

_____

_____

_____

Despite Paul's sage instructions, all too often we make poor choices when it comes to balancing our time budgets, and consequently we end up shortchanging or even eliminating the items that contribute most to our having a balanced lifestyle. And we do so at a very high cost! In our quest to do more and more, we don't make time for important things like spending time alone with God, getting to know Him better. In our rush to get all of our worldly busyness accomplished, we also have a tendency to put off until tomorrow things that need to be done every day, like exercise, if we plan to accomplish our First Place 4 Health goals. For example, we may think to ourselves, *I don't have time for exercise today, so I'll exercise twice as long tomorrow.* Then when tomorrow comes, we're lucky if we exercise at all. Such poor time management obviously is not only bad for our health, but it is also bad for our souls.

We must make wise use of our time by setting priorities. We need to be purposeful about what's important. We need to discipline ourselves to do what has lasting value and is good for us, and we need to set limits on the time we spend doing other things. And when we feel tired or think we still won't get everything important done, we need to remember the words of Isaiah 40:28-29:

> Do you not know? Have you not heard? The LORD is the everlasting God, the Creator of the ends of the earth. He will not grow tired or weary, and his understanding no one can fathom. He gives strength to the weary and increases the power of the weak.

God understands us and what we face every day. He's here to help us, and He's never too busy. We simply have to call on Him. Remember that the race in which we participate is a marathon, not a sprint. We must pace ourselves in order to finish and win the prize God has for us.

Gracious God, teach me to always put into practice what I know will help me to live a balanced lifestyle centered on You and Your Word. I want the cloud of witnesses to see me run my race without faltering at the finish line. Amen.

REFLECTION AND APPLICATION

God, I know that when I obey You, You will help me win the prize I seek and will help me achieve all of my First Place 4 Health goals. Guide me to be firm in my faithfulness to You and to the program. Amen.

Although Jesus knew what awaited Him in Jerusalem, He "resolutely set out for Jerusalem" (Luke 9:51). Jesus was determined to do His Father's will, and in our lives we should exhibit that same sort of fixed purpose, or resolve, if we hope to achieve our goals emotionally, spiritually, mentally and physically. Jesus had a divine appointment in Jerusalem, and it was important that He stay on schedule. Jesus knew what He had been sent to accomplish, and He was determined to do it.

Just as God had inscribed on His Son's heart a plan that would put Jesus in Jerusalem at the time of the Passover feast, so too God has placed a plan in your heart! And just as nothing—absolutely nothing—was going to keep Jesus from doing His Father's will, so too should you be so determined to follow through with God's plan for you.

It is your Father's will that you make the necessary preparations and take the needed steps that will bring you to where He wants you to be—and that you arrive at your destination in keeping with His good and perfect timing. Resolutely setting out is what distinguishes dreams from goals! We dream of achieving many things, but only the things we resolutely set out to accomplish will become reality.

What concrete steps are you taking that show you have resolutely set out to reach your desired destination in the First Place 4 Health program?

_____

_____

_____

_____

_____

_____

_____

What concrete steps are you taking that show you have resolutely set out to reach the desired destination (eternal life) that God has for you?

_____

_____

_____

_____

_____

There is one more step you need to take in order to resolutely set out to reach your goals: Proverbs 16:3 says that you should "commit to the LORD whatever you do, and your plans will succeed." Have you truly committed your plans and goals to God? Who is in control? Are you willing to stay the course when times get rough or when things don't go exactly as *you* had planned? Are you doing your part?

What is it that you still need to do in order to fully commit your plans to God?

_____

_____

_____

_____

_____

Spend time today committing to God your First Place 4 Health plans and goals, and then resolutely set out on the journey. With God's help you will succeed. He is with you to bless you!

Loving God, I commit to You all the goals and plans I have made, and I resolve to do my part on my journey to achieve all of my goals. Thank You for Your presence beside me as I walk. Remind me that Jesus is the model I need to copy. I am so grateful for Your love and guidance in all that I do. Amen.

Group Prayer Requests

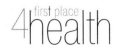

Today's Date: _____

Name	Request

Results

_____

_____

_____

_____

_____

_____

join with others for success

SCRIPTURE MEMORY VERSE

*Let the word of Christ dwell in you richly as you teach and admonish
one another with all wisdom, and as you sing psalms, hymns and spiritual
songs with gratitude in your hearts to God.*

COLOSSIANS 3:16

At the end of Joshua 21, we read about the end of the military opera-
tions in which the nation of Israel had taken part in order to inhabit the
land that the Lord had promised to their forefathers. The Lord had been
steadfast in His love and faithfulness to His Chosen People. Not one of
the covenant promises that the Lord God Almighty had made to their
ancestors had gone unfulfilled:

> So the LORD gave Israel all the land he had sworn to give their
> forefathers, and they took possession of it and settled there. The
> LORD gave them rest on every side, just as he had sworn to their
> forefathers. Not one of their enemies withstood them; the LORD
> handed all their enemies over to them. Not one of all the LORD's
> good promises to the house of Israel failed; every one was ful-
> filled (Joshua 21:43-45).

Although the book from which the above quote comes bears the
name of the man chosen by God to lead the children of Israel into the
Promised Land, that conquest was God's working through a community

effort, not the result of one man's efforts. As the Bible aptly reminds us, the promises—and the inheritance—were given "to the house of Israel."

The Lord had indeed been with the Chosen People to bless *them,* with the emphasis on "them." Note the pronouns that are used in the Scripture passage given above: "their," "they" and "them." This was not an inheritance given to one person or to even one tribe. This was an inheritance given to an entire nation—the nation of Israel—and it would be a blessing to "all peoples on earth" (Genesis 12:3).

Last week, we learned about the "great cloud of witnesses" who encourage us and inspire us. And earlier in this study, we learned about the importance of the legacy we are passing on to generations yet to come. This week we will learn about a third group of people who play an important role in our Christian walk and in our First Place 4 Health endeavors: others who are making the journey with us.

Day 1 — STRENGTH AND FELLOWSHIP

Lord God, Your plan and purposes entail my joining with others to accomplish Your plans for me. Thank You for the strength and fellowship provided by my companions on this journey. Amen.

God did not design us to live isolated lives. Read Ecclesiastes 4:8-12. What does a person who works alone think of his or her toil (see verse 8)?

_____

_____

_____

_____

Of what does a loner deprive himself or herself (see verse 8)?

_____

_____

_____

_____

Why is it better to work with someone than to work alone (see verses 9-10)?

_____

_____

_____

_____

_____

What may happen if a person works alone (see verse 10)?

_____

_____

_____

_____

_____

What is even better than two people who work together, and why (see verse 12)?

_____

_____

_____

_____

_____

What are a few specific ways in which joining the First Place 4 Health program is similar to becoming part of "a cord of three strands"?

_____

_____

_____

_____

_____

Gracious God, You invite me to join with others so that I can be stronger
and have good company on my journey to live a balanced lifestyle.
Thank You for always doing what is best for Your people. Amen.

ENCOURAGEMENT

Lord God, You call me to encourage my brothers and sisters in Christ so that none of us will be deceived by Satan's lies. Thank You for those who help me to be the person You created me to be. Amen.

Encouragement from others is only one of the many benefits found in joining with others for success. Read Hebrews 3:13. How often are we to encourage one another, and why?

_____

_____

_____

_____

_____

Look at 2 Corinthians 2:11. What does Satan do to try to discourage us and turn us away from God?

_____

_____

_____

_____

_____

What instruction does Peter give us in 1 Peter 5:8-9?

_____

_____

_____

_____

In what ways is Satan like a lion?

_____

_____

_____

_____

When you feel discouraged, what should you do?

_____

_____

_____

Now turn to Hebrews 10:24-25. How are we to encourage one another?

_____

_____

_____

_____

Why is the act of meeting together encouragement itself?

_____

_____

_____

What are a few specific ways that you can encourage the others in your First Place 4 Health group?

_____

_____

_____

_____

Gracious God, You put people in my life who encourage and strengthen me. Thank You for those who spur me on to love and good deeds. Amen.

BLESSING

Day 3

Dear God, You shower Your blessings on those who assemble together to hear Your Word and learn more about You. Thank You for allowing me to be a grateful recipient of Your bounty. Amen.

All four gospels record Jesus' feeding 5,000 people. Read Luke's account in Luke 9:12-17. Thousands of people had come to a remote place to listen to Jesus teach. When evening began to set in, what did the 12 disciples ask Jesus to do, and what was Jesus' response (see verses 12-13)?

_____

_____

_____

_____

In reply, on what did the disciples focus (see verse 13)?

_____

_____

_____

_____

What resource did the Twelve have that they failed to consider in their calculations?

_____

_____

_____

_____

_____

How did Jesus solve the problem (see verses 16-17)?

_____

_____

_____

_____

What specific thing did Jesus do to indicate the true source of the blessing the crowd was about to receive (see verse 16)?

_____

_____

_____

_____

Read Psalm 67. For whom are God's blessings intended? What response is given for God's blessings?

_____

_____

_____

_____

_____

What are some of the specific blessings you've received by being part of the First Place 4 Health program?

_____

_____

_____

_____

_____

Little is much in Your hands, O Lord. Thank You for placing me in a First Place 4 Health group where I can receive Your abundant blessings and then share them with others. Amen.

LESSONS AND ADMONISHMENT

Day 4

O Lord, guide me to be open to the instruction of others and to admonishment by others when I need it. I don't want to stray away from You and everything You have to give me. Amen.

Our memory verse tells us about another benefit of being part of a group. Write from memory Colossians 3:16.

_____

_____

_____

_____

_____

Why is it so important that the first instruction comes before the others in our memory verse?

_____

_____

_____

How does the First Place 4 Health program prepare us to follow that first instruction?

_____

_____

_____

_____

How can you teach others in your group (how can your contribution to the group be a lesson for someone else)?

_____

_____

_____

_____

What does "admonish" mean? How is admonishment to be handled (see 1 Thessalonians 5:14)?

_____

_____

_____

_____

Why must we be willing to listen to admonishment in regard to our Christian walk as well as to our First Place 4 Health endeavors?

_____

_____

_____

_____

Why should all of our songs to God—even when we're troubled—be sung "with gratitude"?

_____

_____

_____

_____

God of hope, You fill me with joy and peace as I trust in You. Thank You for the companions You've given me who help to teach me and are willing to encourage me on the right path. You fill my life with all good things. Amen.

FAMILY · Day 5

Gracious Father, thank You for allowing me to be part of the great family of God. Your Spirit guarantees me that I am a child of God. Amen.

Just as Joshua and the people he led into the Promised Land were part of a larger body—"the house of Israel"—modern Christians are also part of a larger body—the Body of Christ. Yes, we are individuals, but more importantly, we are part of the great family of God! Read 1 Corinthians 12:12-27. How are we like the parts of a human body (see verses 12-13)?

_____

_____

_____

What specifically makes us all part of the same Body, or family of God (see verse 13)?

_____

_____

_____

_____

Why is each member of the Body important and necessary (see verses 14-20)?

_____

_____

_____

_____

_____

Why should no member of the family look down on or envy any other member (see verses 21-25)?

_____

_____

_____

_____

Why is what happens to one member of the Body so important (see verse 26)?

_____

_____

_____

_____

Although we should each have a personal relationship with God, why should we also build relationships with other members of God's family?

_____

_____

_____

_____

_____

Gracious God, You have placed me in Your family and given me a role to play. Help me to recognize the importance of my function in the Body so that I can join with others to fulfill what You have called us to do. Amen.

REFLECTION AND APPLICATION

*O Lord, You are my strength and my song. Thank You for giving me a
collection of psalms to sing as a means of encouraging myself and others. Amen.*

Our memory verse this week, Colossians 3:16, encourages us to "sing
psalms, hymns and spiritual songs with gratitude in your hearts to God."
And in those words we learn an essential spiritual truth: Prayer and song,
when coupled together, produce a harmony pleasing to God.

Perhaps that truth explains why we see singing intertwined in the
lives of God's people throughout Scripture. The pages of the Bible are
full of instances when people used music to give expression to their
hopes, their faith and their thanks. (For an example in the Old Testament, see the song of Moses and Miriam [Exodus 15:1-21]; for an example in the New Testament, see Mary's song [Luke 1:46-55].) And many
of the early hymns of the Church are still popular today, so God's music is not restricted to time or place. The very ability to sing, even if it's a
bit off-key, is a mark of God's grace. As a matter of fact, our soulful songs
may be our greatest witness to a world that cannot hear the gospel in
any other form.

Learning to sing songs of praise is a wonderful way to recite the time-
honored words of the Bible. Set to music, the Scriptures come alive with
a rhythm and harmony not always possible when the words are read
silently or even when they are read out loud in worship. Research has
shown time and time again that words set to music are easier to memorize and retain. That's why all the First Place 4 Health memory verses in
this Bible study have been set to music and made available for your use.

As we sing psalms, hymns and spiritual songs, not only is our faith
built up at the very moment we give voice to a song, but also we store up
a reserve of inner strength for those times when trouble invites us to sing
a different tune. Having filled our hearts and minds with God's truth,
there will always be a song of praise ready in our hearts and minds—a song
of joy and thanksgiving that we can sing at anytime, in anyplace. Singing
hymns, psalms and spiritual songs reminds us of God's faithfulness and

love. God is our strength and our song; and when we sing of His faithfulness, others listen.

End your reflection time today by singing a psalm, hymn or spiritual song. And remember to sing it with gratitude in your heart to God!

When I sing of Your goodness and grace, O God, I am built up in my faith. Thank You for my voice and my ability to use it in a variety of ways. Thank You too for the gift of music and song. Let my voice always be raised in thanks to You for all Your wonderful promises and the fact that You are faithful to those promises. Amen.

Day 7 REFLECTION AND APPLICATION

In Your wisdom, gracious God, You put me in a First Place 4 Health group that is perfectly suited to my needs. Thank You for making this provision for my spiritual growth. Amen.

On day five of this week's study, we learned about the family of God, which is often referred to as the Body of Christ. In a larger sense, the Body of Christ is the Church universal, and its composition includes all people—from every nation, from every walk of life, and of every color and size—who call Jesus their Savior and Lord. All who have received Jesus as their Lord and Savior are part of the Body of Christ.

Within that broader context, every local church community can be considered a part of the larger Body and can also be considered a smaller version of that larger Body. Members of a local church are brought together by God and called to function as one body. Christ, in His wisdom, gives us spiritual gifts to be used, not for self-glorification, but for the greater good of the body in which God has placed us—both the local body and the universal Body.

What is true of the Church universal, and on a smaller scale true of the local church, also applies to every group of Christians who assemble together in Christ's name. Therefore, your First Place 4 Health group is an even smaller version of the Body of Christ. You were placed in this particular group, at this particular time in salvation history, because you have something that the group needs—and every other person in the group has something you need. We are all members of the Body—and we need one another!

In what way do you help the local Body of Christ?

_____

_____

_____

_____

_____

Now think of the people in your First Place 4 Health group. Beside the name of each individual, note what that person has to offer the group and how that person is a blessing to the group. Be sure to list yourself, too.

_____

_____

_____

_____

_____

Gracious God, I am blessed to be a blessing. You have given me gifts and talents to use to build up the Body of Christ. Thank You for including me in Your great plan and purpose. Amen.

Group Prayer Requests

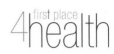

Today's Date: _____

Name	Request

Results

_____

_____

_____

_____

_____

_____

choose whom
you will serve

SCRIPTURE MEMORY VERSE
*Those who know your name will trust in you, for you, LORD,
have never forsaken those who seek you.*
PSALM 9:10

When all of the tribes had taken possession of the portion of land that was their promised inheritance, God gave His people rest from all their enemies—the gift of peace that allowed them to enjoy the other good things He had given them. By now Joshua was "old and well advanced in years," and he knew it would soon be time for him to leave the people he had faithfully led for many years (Joshua 23:1). However, he knew that there was one more thing that had to be done before he went "the way of all the earth" (Joshua 23:14). He summoned all the leaders of Israel to meet with him so that he could remind them of their responsibilities, both to God and to the people they were called to govern. In his farewell speech, Joshua reminded them of all the amazing things God had done for Israel—and what they must do if they hoped to remain in God's favor:

> I am old and well advanced in years. You yourselves have seen everything the LORD your God has done to all these nations for your sake; it was the LORD your God who fought for you. Be very strong; be careful to obey all that is written in the Book of the Law of Moses, without turning aside to the right or to the left. The LORD has driven out before you great and powerful nations;

to this day no one has been able to withstand you. One of you routs a thousand, because the LORD your God fights for you, just as he promised (Joshua 23:2-3,6,9-10).

In addition to admonishing the leaders to remember how their faithful God had fought for Israel and how He had given them this good land as their inheritance, Joshua reminded them of another important truth. Just as God had fulfilled all His good promises, so too God would do what He had sworn to do if the people turned away from Him to serve false gods. Therefore, it was imperative that the leaders encourage the people to hold fast to the Lord, to cling to Him and not be enticed to bow down to and serve other gods. Joshua summed up his admonition to remain faithful with these words: "So be very careful to love the LORD your God" (Joshua 23:11).

Like Israel of old, we, too, are to hold fast to the Lord. We must be careful to love our God and we must not worship and serve the things of this world. God is our life, and keeping Him first in all things is our greatest responsibility.

Day 1 LOVE EACH OTHER

Sovereign Lord, thank You for calling me to be part of Your great family here on earth. How blessed I am to be among those who have placed their trust in You. Amen.

God, who chooses us to be members of the Body of Christ, places us exactly where He wants us to be. Read John 15:12-17. What did Jesus command His disciples to do (see verses 12,17)?

_____

_____

_____

_____

What did Jesus say was the greatest example of following this command, and how did Jesus model it (see verse 13)?

_____

_____

_____

_____

_____

Why are we able to love others (see verses 14-16; see also 1 John 4:19)?

_____

_____

_____

Now turn to 1 John 4:15-21. According to John, what is the source of human love (see verses 15-16)?

_____

_____

_____

_____

If we ever become fearful, what should we do (see verses 17-18)?

_____

_____

_____

_____

What does how we treat others show the rest of the world (see verses 20-21)?

_____

_____

_____

_____

Although we will probably not ever be asked to make the same sacrifice as Jesus, in what ways can we sacrifice in order to show love to someone?

_____

_____

_____

_____

_____

> *Gracious God, You are love and all that You do is loving. Let Your love shine through me to others. I want to show the world the great God I serve. Teach me to rely on Your love and strength so that I never shy away from loving others. Amen.*

Day 2 **SERVE ONLY GOD**

Loving Lord, I can either love and serve You with all my heart, mind, soul and strength; or I can give my devotion to false gods—I can't do both. Thank You for giving me the freedom to choose, and guide me to always choose to serve only You. Amen.

In his final address to the tribes of Israel, Joshua spoke about the people renewing their covenant with God. Read Joshua 24:2-27. Of what were the people reminded (see verses 2-13)?

_____

_____

_____

_____

What did Joshua say that the people should do (see verse 14)?

_____

_____

_____

_____

What three options were the people given (see verses 14-15)?

1. _____
2. _____
3. _____

What was Joshua's choice (see verse 15)?

_____
_____
_____
_____

What did the people choose to do, and why (see verses 16-18)?

_____
_____
_____
_____

What did Joshua tell the people to do, and why was doing that important (see verse 23)?

_____
_____
_____
_____

What purpose did the stone serve, and why was this important (see verses 26-27)?

_____
_____
_____
_____

What are some of the idols that people worship today?

_____

_____

_____

_____

_____

Why should they be "thrown away"?

_____

_____

_____

_____

_____

Thank You, Lord God Almighty, for giving me the freedom to make a choice about whom I will serve. I choose to serve only You, for I know that You are the true foundation of every aspect of my life. And I will make the same choice every day! Amen.

Day 3 — TRUST ONLY GOD

Because I know Your name, O Lord, I will trust in You. All that You have promised Your people, You will do! You are steadfast and faithful, and I am grateful. Amen.

Our great God is deserving and worthy of the trust we are called to give Him in this week's memory verse. From memory, write Psalm 9:10.

_____

_____

_____

_____

_____

_____

According to the following passages, what does God do for those who trust in Him?

1 Chronicles 5:20: _____

Psalm 37:3-6: _____

Psalm 115:9-11: _____

Proverbs 29:25: _____

Isaiah 26:3: _____

Turn to John 14:1. According to Jesus, what should a person do when he or she feels troubled?

_____

_____

_____

_____

Now look at Habakkuk 2:18. What is the difference between the idols the world suggests we worship and the God we should worship?

_____

_____

_____

_____

Briefly describe what happened during a time when you relied on your own strength, rather than trusting God.

_____

_____

_____

_____

Lord God, You call me to trust in You. Help me to be faithful and not turn to idols of this world. It is You who are strong and it is You who are reliable. Thank You for blessing me when I trust in You only. Amen.

Day
4

SEEK GOD

Because I know Your name, O Lord, I will trust in You. You are steadfast and faithful, and I will continue to seek You all my days. Amen.

This week's memory verse tells us not only to trust God but also to seek God. Read Psalm 14:1-3. Why are those who don't believe in God either foolish or corrupt?

_____

_____

_____

_____

_____

For what does God look (see verse 2)?

_____

_____

_____

_____

Turn to Psalm 63:1-5. How does David describe his need to be close to God (see verse 1)?

_____

_____

_____

_____

_____

What did David know about God that would satisfy him (see verses 2-3)?

_____

_____

_____

_____

_____

What did David plan to do because He knew God (see verse 4)?

_____

_____

_____

_____

_____

What did David expect to happen (see verse 5)?

_____

_____

_____

_____

What did the writer of Hebrews say will happen to those who seek God (see Hebrews 11:6)?

_____

_____

_____

_____

What are a couple of ways that you can actively seek God?

_____

_____

_____

_____

_____

Thank You, O Lord, for encouraging me to seek You so that You can build me up and strengthen my faith. Keep me ever mindful of Your love and presence. Only You can truly satisfy. Amen.

BE A FAITHFUL SERVANT

Lord God, I know the day will come when I stand before You to give an accounting of how I have managed my affairs. Merciful Father, I pray for the grace to be found faithful. Amen.

Being prepared to account for the choices we have made is a concept most of us would rather not think about, but think about it we must. Turn to Romans 14:10-12. What will all of us one day have to do?

_____

_____

_____

_____

Turn to Romans 8:1-4. What is one thing that believers will never face (see verse 1)?

_____

_____

_____

_____

What did Jesus do for all those who believe in Him, and how did that free us (see verses 2-3)?

_____

_____

_____

_____

How are we supposed to live (see verse 4)?

_____

_____

_____

_____

Read Matthew 25:14-30, the parable of the talents. What did the master give to each servant, and what did each servant do with what he had been given (see verses 14-18)?

_____

_____

_____

_____

When the master returned home, what was his reaction to what the first two servants had done with what they had been given (see verses 19-23)?

_____

_____

_____

_____

What was the master's reaction to what the third servant had done with what he had been given (see verses 24-30)?

_____

_____

_____

_____

Which of the three servants best represents what you have done with your talents? Why?

_____

_____

_____

_____

Thank You, Lord, for reminding me that I will one day stand before
You to give an account of what I have done with what You have given me.
Teach me to be a faithful steward of Your blessings. I want to hear You
say to me, "Well done, good and faithful servant!" Amen.

REFLECTION AND APPLICATION

Merciful God, I know that You are a loving Father who wants only the best for me. Let me lean on You so that I can more confidently use Your gifts so that I am faithful to Your plans for me. Amen.

Accountability partners and accountability groups help us achieve positive lifestyle changes. Not only do these important people provide advice and encouragement to help us in our daily walk with God, but they also help keep us honest with ourselves. They hold us accountable as we attempt to implement the small daily changes that allow us to persevere in our efforts to realize our goals and plans. (If you haven't already done so, take time now to read about accountability and support in the *First Place 4 Health Member's Guide* [see the first two chapters in section 3].)

Yet as important as these partners are in our Christian faith-journey, we can never forget that they only serve as representatives of the One to whom all believers are ultimately accountable. They remind us that we are stewards and that we have a Master who will someday return to settle accounts with us.

Perhaps part of our confusion when we contemplate this thing called accountability comes from our misunderstanding of the word "steward" and of the master/steward relationship that is the basis of biblical stewardship. Many people today think of a steward as a lowly servant-slave. But in Jesus' day, a steward was not a menial slave. A steward was in a noble position that involved oversight of all the master's possessions and business ventures and included the prudent management of time, energy, material resources, gifts, physical abilities, and the diligent supervision of all the people and resources under the steward's authority.

The same is true today. Being a steward is a high calling and a noble position that is reserved for those who have been created, sustained, saved and called to do the good works the Master has planned in advance for them to do.

When we practice living a life that is balanced emotionally, spiritually, mentally and physically, we are being faithful stewards of the earthly bodies God has entrusted to us as vehicles for doing His work here on earth. When we do good deeds with what God has given us, we show that our faith is alive and that we are being good stewards of God's grace.

Unfortunately, we sometimes forget that the motive behind what we do must be sincere and come naturally from a close relationship with God. The relationship between each of us (stewards) and the Master is not to be taken lightly. Our motives behind whatever we do must be pure, "for the LORD searches every heart and understands every motive behind the thoughts" (1 Chronicles 28:9). Do anything superficially or only for the sake of appearance, and God will know it. An empty gesture is still an empty gesture, no matter the reason for it.

Think about the motives you had for doing some of the things you've done in the past. Have your motives always been pure? Have you ever done anything out of spite? Have you ever rushed to be ahead of someone because you were in a hurry and assumed the other person wasn't? Would you feel comfortable bringing to the light the reasons for everything you've done?

As you conclude today's reflection, what is one thing you need to work on so that your motives are pure?

_____

_____

_____

_____

_____

Lord God, You call me to have a loving relationship with You.
Help me to be honest and pure of heart so that I happily and sincerely
steward all that You have given me. I have heard Your voice, and I
want to serve only You in grateful obedience. Amen.

Day
7

REFLECTION AND APPLICATION

Gracious God, You have given me everything I need to live a life of godliness. Thank You for sending the right people into my life at just the right time. I know that they will help me as I choose to serve only You. Amen.

In each of our lives, there is an important "principle of three" that is part of our spiritual growth. Each of us needs to have in our lives a Paul, a Barnabas and a Timothy. We need a Paul to teach us in the faith, a Barnabas to journey alongside us and encourage us in the faith, and a Timothy whom we nurture and train in the faith. In the kingdom of God we are all called to be disciples, encouragers and teachers—believers who do not stop seeking knowledge of the Lord on this side of heaven. Paul, Barnabas and Timothy relationships give us the balance and harmony necessary for Christian maturity.

Paul was a mentor to a great many people. He was the first apostle to teach the Gentiles, and the book of Acts tells about all of his missionary journeys to spread the gospel to others. We need to find and be a disciple of a Paul who can be a mentor to us, someone who can teach us, someone we can listen to and observe, whose example we can follow as we grow in our faith.

Barnabas's name makes clear why we should pursue having a Barnabas in our lives: His name means "Son of Encouragement" (Acts 4:36). We all need someone to support us and encourage us to never give up our goals, both on our Christian walk and on our First Place 4 Health journey. Barnabas was the apostle who supported Paul when Paul returned from preaching to the Gentiles, and he traveled with Paul on many of his missions. We all need a champion in our corner, urging us on and giving us a hand when needed, a companion who believes that our abilities can take us wherever we need to go.

Timothy was like a brother to Paul, and Paul trained Timothy, his devoted follower. We all need a Timothy, someone to whom we can pass on our knowledge, with whom we in turn share our faith. Each of us should be able to say what John wrote to Gaius: "I have no greater joy than to hear that my children are walking in the truth" (3 John 4). By influencing an-other person—by our support and encouragement, by our teaching and modeling—we also continue to learn and grow. And as we hold another person accountable, we ourselves become more accountable.

Look at your earthly relationships. Who is your Paul, your Barnabas and your Timothy? (If you lack any of these, ask God to bring people into your life who will fill each of these vital roles.)

My Paul is: _____

My Barnabas is:_____

My Timothy is: _____

Dear God, thank You for bringing me a Paul to teach me, a Barnabas to encourage me, and a Timothy who I can mentor as I continue to be built up in my faith. You indeed know what I need before I even ask. Your love knows no bounds, and I want Your love to shine through me to others so that they too will choose to serve only You. Amen.

Group Prayer Requests

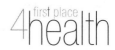

Today's Date: _____

Name	Request

Results

_____

_____

_____

_____

_____

recognize God's authority and power

SCRIPTURE MEMORY VERSE

That at the name of Jesus every knee should bow, in heaven and on earth and under the earth, and every tongue confess that Jesus Christ is Lord, to the glory of God the Father.

PHILIPPIANS 2:10-11

Some 40 years before Joshua led God's people into the Promised Land, Moses had gone to Pharaoh with these words: "This is what the LORD, the God of the Hebrews, says: 'Let my people go, so that they may worship me'" (Exodus 9:1).

But Pharaoh's heart was hard. It was only after several signs, many wonders and a series of plagues that Pharaoh relented and agreed to let God's people go. Then began the Exodus: God led the children of Israel out of Egypt, through the Red Sea, 40 years in the desert and then safely to the land God had promised to give their ancestors. Even though the children of Israel were occasionally stiff-necked and rebellious, God was faithful to His covenant promise to deliver them from the bondage of Egypt and keep them as His own treasured possession.

In the Old Testament, God's ultimate display of power and might was the raising of this "dead" nation Israel. Israel had been in captivity, enslaved by the cruel taskmasters in Egypt, and God delivered them. As the Scriptures repeat over and over again: "You brought your people Israel out of Egypt with signs and wonders, by a mighty hand and an outstretched arm and with great terror" (Jeremiah 32:21).

The Scriptures also repeat over and over the command to remember well what God has done for you, to recall how with might and power the Lord freed His people and brought them to a land overflowing with milk and honey (see, for example, Deuteronomy 7:18). Along with the perpetual call to remembrance often came the same question: "I am the LORD, the God of all mankind. Is anything too hard for me?" (Jeremiah 32:27).

Today, the same Lord that brought Israel out of captivity; the same Lord that sustained His Chosen People in the wilderness; the same Lord that had Joshua lead the Israelites into the Promised Land that was their inheritance assures us that His authority and power have not changed and will not change. We can successfully complete our First Place 4 Health journeys and we can complete our faith journeys, because everything is under the authority of God. God is in control, and nothing is too hard for Him.

Day 1 — GOD'S RESURRECTION POWER

Lord God, nothing is too hard for You. Not one of the problems or situations I face today is a match for Your might and power. Thank You for being by my side. Amen.

Just as the raising up of a "dead" nation is the supreme example of God's power found in the Old Testament, so too the resurrection of Jesus Christ from the dead is the supreme example of God's power found in the New Testament. Just as Israel was in captivity and enslaved by the cruel taskmasters in Egypt before God delivered them, so too we were in captivity before Christ delivered us! Read Ephesians 2:1-7. In what respect were we dead (see verses 1-3)?

_____

_____

_____

_____

_____

Why did God save us (see verse 4)?

How did God make us alive (see verse 5)?

Because we are made alive with Christ, what kind of life can we enjoy (see verses 6-7)?

According to John 11:25, how did Jesus describe Himself and His power?

How would you describe resurrection life for the believer?

Gracious God, Your power is so great that You raise the dead. I am thankful that You are rich in love, that by grace You have saved me, that You forgive my sins and that You will one day raise me to live with You. Amen.

JESUS' ULTIMATE POWER

*Lamb of God, thank You for becoming the perfect sacrifice for my sins.
I did nothing to deserve Your mercy and favor. Your grace, and Your
grace alone, saved me. Amen.*

Not only did the mighty power of God raise Jesus from the dead, but
that same resurrection power also now lives in all who have confessed
Jesus as Savior and Lord! Read Paul's words in Ephesians 1:18-23. What
is the inheritance of all believers (see verse 18)?

_____

_____

_____

_____

What is available for all believers (see verse 19)?

_____

_____

_____

_____

Where did God place Jesus after He raised Him from the dead (see verses
20-21)?

_____

_____

_____

_____

Over what does Jesus rule (see verses 22-23)?

_____

_____

_____

_____

Turn to John 10:29-30. In addition to being the Shepherd of His people, what did Jesus describe Himself as being?

_____

_____

_____

_____

Who do you say Jesus is?

_____

_____

_____

_____

(If you are not sure how to answer the question above, please talk to your First Place 4 Health group leader or other trusted Christian leader about why your answer to the question is so important.)

> *Lord God, I know that You are the ultimate power, and Your might*
> *is beyond even what I can imagine it to be. Thank You for using Your*
> *power for my benefit. Amen.*

OUR POWER SOURCE   Day 3

> *Thank You, God, that You give us access to Your power through*
> *the Holy Spirit. Amen.*

The same power that raised Jesus from the dead lives in us. Look at Colossians 1:9-12. What did Paul want believers to have (see verses 9-10)?

_____

_____

_____

_____

_____

What is the source of our power to do what is right (see verse 11)?

_____

_____

_____

_____

_____

Turn to Acts 1:8. When do we receive the power?

_____

_____

_____

_____

Now read John 16:12-15. What did Jesus say this power source would do for us (see verse 13)?

_____

_____

_____

_____

Why does the power source do this for us (see verse 14)?

_____

_____

_____

_____

What are a few of the ways that the world tries to turn us away from the true source of power?

_____

_____

_____

_____

What are a few specific ways that believers can show that the true source of power is working in their lives?

_____

_____

_____

_____

_____

Thank You, gracious Father, for giving me the power I need to do what is right. Thank You for guiding me to live in and by the truth. Teach me to listen to Your voice and follow Your lead. Amen.

JESUS' EXAMPLE

Day 4

Jesus, You came to show me the love and power of the Father, even as You came to show me how to live a life pleasing to Him. Today I will look to You as my example. Amen.

Jesus is our example of depending on the power of God. Read Hebrews 5:8-9. What was the result of Jesus' obedience?

_____

_____

_____

_____

_____

According to John 5:19,30, on whom did Jesus rely?

_____

_____

_____

_____

Now look at Matthew 26:36-42. Jesus prayed to God and asked God to do what (see verse 39)?

_____

_____

_____

What did Jesus choose to do (see verses 39,42)?

_____

_____

_____

Jesus prayed often (see Matthew 19:13; Mark 1:35; Luke 5:16; 6:12; 9:18; 11:1). Why do you think Jesus prayed to God?

_____

_____

_____

_____

Read Luke 11:1. How did the disciples respond to Jesus' habit of prayer?

_____

_____

_____

How do you incorporate prayer into your daily life?

_____

_____

_____

_____

_My Lord and my God, it is my desire to always do Your will. Help me
to look to You throughout my day so that I always know what I should do.
I want to follow the example of Jesus and be obedient. Amen._

JESUS' NAME

Dear Father, I confess that Jesus is my Lord, and I praise You for what Your amazing power has done for me. Amen.

This week's memory verse tells us about a glorious day yet to come. From memory, write Philippians 2:10-11.

_____

_____

_____

_____

_____

Who exactly will one day recognize the authority and power of Jesus?

_____

_____

_____

_____

What will that recognition cause to happen?

_____

_____

_____

_____

_____

Look at Philippians 2:9. What authority did God give the name of Jesus?

_____

_____

_____

_____

According to John 14:13-14, under what circumstance will Jesus do something for us?

_____

_____

_____

_____

According to what Peter told the crowd at Pentecost, what are the results of repentance and being baptized (see Acts 2:38)?

_____

_____

_____

_____

Turn to Acts 3:1-7. What did Peter say when he healed the beggar (see verse 6)? What does this tell you about the source of the beggar's healing?

_____

_____

_____

_____

Why do you think that even when we pray "in the name of Jesus," the result isn't always what _we_ want?

_____

_____

_____

_____

_____

Dear Jesus, You have promised that You will do what I ask, if I ask in Your name. Help me to keep my motives for asking pure, and guide me to see that You will give me only good things—which aren't always the same as that for which I have asked. Amen.

REFLECTION AND APPLICATION

Father, You are my Good Shepherd. You lead me in right paths
for Your name's sake. How grateful I am that I am a sheep in
Your pasture and You are my Lord. Amen.

Were we asked to live the Christian life in our own strength and power, we would all be lost. However, Jesus did not leave us as orphans. Just as the Lord had been with Joshua and the Israelites to bless them, so too by the power of the Holy Spirit our Lord is with us! He fights for us, He protects us, He provides for us, and He encourages us as He leads and guides us. He is our "good shepherd" (John 10:11), our "great Shepherd" (Hebrews 13:20) and our "Chief Shepherd" (1 Peter 5:4).

Probably no other psalm in the Bible states the relationship between God as a shepherd and His followers as His sheep so clearly as Psalm 23. Penned by David—a shepherd himself at one time—Psalm 23 is a sort of summary description of how God's presence, power, protection and provision belong to all believers. As you read through this psalm, consider each line carefully: Think about what God provides for us, how He heals and revives us, and how He guides us (and why He does it). And don't forget that He can even still the waters, if a storm comes up. As sheep, all we need to do is follow His lead. With God as our Shepherd, we have no reason to be scared, even though we may have troubles in this life and we may feel attacked by others. Remind yourself of what God will do for us, how He reassures us and protects us, and what our final destination will be.

Which of our Shepherd's benefits are you most in need of today? Do you need rest, tranquility, restoration, guidance, protection, provision, purpose, mercy, assurance?

The Good Shepherd has promised that you will have everything you need! As you review what your Shepherd promises to do for you, write a prayer telling Him how you need His help today. Remember to be specific and to end your prayer by thanking your Good Shepherd for being with you.

_____

_____

_____

_____

Good Shepherd, show me how I can stay safely in Your flock and not be distracted by anything or anyone pretending to offer greener pastures. Only You have the power to provide what I need. Amen.

Day 7 — REFLECTION AND APPLICATION

Loving Lord, help me to surround myself with those who recognize Your authority and power. Let my life be an example to others, and help me to choose friends who will help me get to know You better. Amen.

We need to select our inner circle from among those who hear the Word of God and put it into practice. Only those who trust in the name of Jesus can encourage our faith, support us and help us up when we falter or fall. Only those who know God's promises and trust in His faithfulness can remind us of the Lord's steadfast love when we find ourselves questioning our faith, worried about reaching our goals to live a balanced lifestyle, or concerned about some problem we're facing. Only those who recognize God's authority and power are able to guide us to do what is right in God's eyes and help us to live a balanced lifestyle. According to the Bible:

> A righteous man is cautious in friendship, but the way of the wicked leads them astray (Proverbs 12:26).

> He who walks with the wise grows wise, but a companion of fools suffers harm (Proverbs 13:20).

A friend loves at all times, and a brother is born for adversity (Proverbs 17:17).

Do not make friends with a hot-tempered man, do not associate with one easily angered, or you may learn his ways and get yourself ensnared (Proverbs 22:24-25).

Wounds from a friend can be trusted, but an enemy multiplies kisses. . . . Perfume and incense bring joy to the heart, and the pleasantness of one's friend springs from his earnest counsel. . . . As iron sharpens iron, so one man sharpens another (Proverbs 27:6,9,17).

Do not be misled: "Bad company corrupts good character" (1 Corinthians 15:33).

The friends with whom we spend our time can either help us or hurt us. They can either sharpen our abilities or dull our senses. They can help us reach up to God or drag us down to Satan. They can help us be free to reap the rewards of heaven or tie us down to this world.

Think about the people who are in your closest circle of friends (outside of your immediate family). Are they people who know the Lord and can encourage you to put your trust in Him? List the names of the friends with whom you spend the most time. How does each of them help you know God better?

Spend the rest of your quiet time today thanking God for friends who strengthen, comfort and encourage you in your faith. Consider writing a note to each of the people, whose names you listed above, thanking them for encouraging you to remain steadfast in your love for the Lord.

All-powerful God, thank You for bringing men and women into my life who will help me to get to know You better. When I am weary, I will remember their prayers and their examples, and I will be strong and courageous. Amen.

Group Prayer Requests

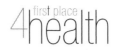

Today's Date: _____

Name	Request

Results

_____

_____

_____

_____

_____

_____

focus on your ultimate goal

SCRIPTURE MEMORY VERSE

The LORD your God is with you, he is mighty to save. He will take great delight in you, he will quiet you with his love, he will rejoice over you with singing.
ZEPHANIAH 3:17

As we have journeyed with Joshua and God's people across the Jordan River into the Promised Land, we have seen the steadfast love and faithfulness of God displayed in amazing ways—just as God had promised Joshua at the start of the journey: God led the Israelites to conquer cities, defeat enemies, and take possession of the land God had promised them as their inheritance. We have briefly looked at the lives of men and women who were part of God's covenant community—some who were faithful and some who were not! We have seen the blessings of obedience and the consequences of sin.

In the book of Hebrews, we learn an amazing thing about the faithful people whose stories we have read—stories given to us as examples to follow:

All these people were still living by faith when they died. They did not receive the things promised; they only saw them and welcomed them from a distance. And they admitted that they were aliens and strangers on earth. People who say such things show that they are looking for a country of their own. If they had been thinking of the country they had left, they would have had opportunity to return. Instead, they were longing for a better country—a heavenly one. Therefore God is not ashamed to be called their God, for he has prepared a city for them (Hebrews 11:13-16).

All the saints who have gone before us were "longing for a better country—a heavenly one." Regardless of what was happening around them, these faithful people were focusing on the ultimate goal, intent on spending eternity with God Almighty who was with them to bless them.

Day 1

LOOK AHEAD

How thankful I am, gracious God, that You are with me to bless me. Because I am focused on the goal and not on my present circumstances, I can put my trust in You. Amen.

The people that Moses led out of Egypt did not always focus on the goal ahead of them. According to the following passages, about what did the people complain?

Exodus 16:1-3: _____

Exodus 17:1-3: _____

Numbers 11:1-6: _____

Numbers 14:1-4: _____

Numbers 20:1-5: _____

With what did the people usually compare their situation?

_____

_____

_____

_____

_____

What did the people forget?

_____

_____

_____

Read Numbers 14:26-35. What was God's response to the repeated complaints of the Israelites in the desert?

_____

_____

_____

What do you think is the largest disadvantage of dwelling on the past?

_____

_____

_____

Briefly describe a time when dwelling on something in the past prevented you from moving forward toward your First Place 4 Health goals.

_____

_____

_____

*God, forgive me for the times I have lost sight of my First Place 4 Health goals
and my goal to be with You in heaven. Guide me to keep my eyes on You and
the true goal ahead, and help me to live in grateful obedience. Amen.*

PRAISE GOD

Day 2

*You, O Lord, are a God who delights in those who delight in You. Thank You
for giving me a grateful heart to replace the grumbling heart that sometimes
threatens to separate me from Your blessing. Amen.*

In direct opposition to those who grumble and complain and feel deprived are those who delight in the Lord who also delights in them, as our memory verse for this week points out. From memory, write out the words of Zephaniah 3:17.

_____

_____

_____

_____

What are the five truths about God in the memory verse?

1. God _____

2. God _____

3. God _____

4. God _____

5. God _____

Let's look at the context of this verse, Zephaniah 3:1-16. What was wrong with the people who were in power in Jerusalem (see verses 1-4)?

_____

_____

_____

_____

What warning did God give that the people in Jerusalem ignored (see verses 6-7)?

_____

_____

_____

What did God say would happen to the people (see verses 8-13)?

_____

_____

_____

_____

Who does God plan to protect (see verses 12-13)?

_____

_____

_____

Why did Zephaniah say that the Israelites would be happy (see verse 15)?

_____

_____

_____

Now turn to Psalm 149:1-5. Why can we delight in God, just as He delights in us? How can we show our delight?

_____

_____

_____

I praise and thank You, marvelous Lord, for being with me
to bless me. I want to make music to praise You, and I want to
hear Your voice raised in song over me. Amen.

ACCEPT DISCIPLINE

Day 3

Loving God, I'm glad that I am one of Your children, but like any other child,
I'm not fond of being disciplined. I know, though, that any discipline You give
me is really for my own good and that it will benefit me. Amen.

Like a human father, our Father in heaven trains us to be more and more like His Son. And part of our upbringing includes correcting or disciplining us when we go astray. Read Romans 8:16. What are we to God?

_____

_____

_____

Now turn to Hebrews 12:5-11. Who does God discipline (see verses 5-6; see also Proverbs 3:11-12)?

_____

_____

_____

_____

Why does God discipline us (see verse 10)?

_____

_____

_____

_____

What does discipline produce (see verse 11)?

_____

_____

_____

_____

Read Psalm 94:12, what will happen to the person who God disciplines?

_____

_____

_____

_____

Why should we accept and even welcome being disciplined by God?

_____

_____

_____

_____

Loving, ever-present Father, help me to learn from those times I need to be disciplined by You so that I repent and turn back to You. Amen.

GAIN WISDOM

*Patient and perfect Teacher, as I meditate on Your truth, help me
to apply it to my life in meaningful ways. Give me the wisdom I need
to grow in my faith. Amen.*

A person who has wisdom is not someone who has a lot of knowledge—
a lot of facts and figures. According to Psalm 111:10, what is the beginning of wisdom?

_____

_____

_____

_____

_____

According to Deuteronomy 4:5-7, how were the Chosen People to show
to the world that they were wise?

_____

_____

_____

_____

_____

Turn to James 1:5. What will God do when we ask Him for wisdom?

_____

_____

_____

_____

Now turn to James 3:13-18. How does a person who is wise act?

_____

_____

_____

_____

What are a few examples of "earthly, unspiritual" wisdom (verse 15)?

_____

_____

_____

_____

Why is true wisdom divine (see verse 17)?

_____

_____

_____

_____

What are a few specific ways that we can grow "in wisdom . . . and in favor with God" (Luke 2:52)?

_____

_____

_____

_____

Gracious God, I need to be wise so that I follow Your ways, rather than following anything the world suggests is the way to be wise. Thank You for giving me Your Word so that I can read about You and what You desire. Grant me the wisdom I need to be like Your Son in every way. Amen.

Day 5 IMAGINE THE FUTURE

Lord God, You are faithful to lead me along right paths. As I focus on my ultimate goal, You allow me to achieve benchmarks that give me hope and encouragement to continue my journey with You. Amen.

As we read about Joshua and his leading of the Chosen People, we learned that God fulfilled His promise to bring His Chosen People to the Promised Land. We have a similar promise from God. Read 1 John

5:13. What is the "Promised Land" that God has promised all believers in Jesus; what is our certain future?

_____

_____

_____

_____

Read Revelation 21:1-4. After God's final judgment, what will appear (see verses 1-2)?

_____

_____

_____

_____

Where will God be (see verse 3)?

_____

_____

_____

_____

What will be missing from this new place (see verse 4)?

_____

_____

_____

_____

Now read Revelation 21:11-25. Although what he saw was unearthly, John had to describe this new place in terms he and his readers would know and understand. To what did John compare what he saw?

_____

_____

_____

Turn to John 14:2-4. What are three things that Jesus told believers about heaven?

1. _____

2. _____

3. _____

According to Philippians 1:6, why should we never doubt God's work in our lives and our future?

_____

_____

_____

_____

Gracious God, thank You for preparing for me a place so grand that human words cannot really describe it. You are the One who always finishes His work, and You have indeed begun a mighty work in me. Amen.

Day 6 — REFLECTION AND APPLICATION

Gracious God, I cannot see the future. I do not see all the twists and turns in the road ahead of me. Yet I know I can walk forward with confidence, for You are with me. Amen.

Although we like to think of our life journeys as straight and level paths, for most of us life is more like a series of switchback trails, potholed walkways, dead-end byways and meandering routes going up the side of a steep mountain. We set our goal and begin the climb, but at times the correct path is difficult to follow. We are always in danger of losing our direction and our footing. Sometimes we try a shortcut that promises to be the easy way but in the end leads either nowhere or back where we started. How do we keep from losing heart as we work our way through the maze of twists and turns on our life journeys?

The first thing we each do is to begin our journey with the end in mind: We keep our focus on the goal, not on our situation or the things happening around us. Our ultimate goal is eternal life with God, so that is where we keep our focus.

Then we consult a map. The best map to eternal life is God's Word. It tells us everything we need to know to reach our goal: "Your word is a lamp to my feet and a light for my path" (Psalm 119:105). When we need to shed some light on a subject, on a decision we need to make, on the way we should go, we need to look at God's Word.

Every once in a while, we also need to look up and evaluate where we are: Are we still going in the right direction? Do we need to backtrack because we've been distracted and have drifted off the path? Are we making progress, or going around in circles? Are we still focusing on the goal?

If we're stuck for some reason and are having trouble moving ahead, we need to consult someone more experienced than we are; someone in the First Place 4 Health group, our pastor or a more mature Christian may be able to help us out and encourage us in the way we should go. And if not, they will likely be able to suggest the name of a Christian professional who can help us with a particular problem that's holding us back.

Remember the words of Jesus: "Enter through the narrow gate. For wide is the gate and broad is the road that leads to destruction, and many enter through it. But small is the gate and narrow the road that leads to life, and only a few find it" (Matthew 7:13-14). The only way to eternal life is through Christ—the narrow gate—and the only way to do that is to walk with God.

Spend a few minutes thinking about where you are on your life journey with God. Where is your focus? Have you been distracted lately? Do you thank God daily for His giving us a way to eternal life?

_____

_____

_____

_____

Where are you on your journey? (At a dead-end? On a switchback? On a meandering walkway? On a straight path? In a pothole?) What is your plan to head in the right direction?

_____

_____

_____

_____

Thank You, merciful God, for giving me the goal of eternal life. When I practice what I learn from reading Your Word, I usually manage to stay on the straight and narrow. But when I seem to lose my way, please shine Your light on the way I should go. I thank You and praise You for all that You do for me and in me. Amen.

Day 7

REFLECTION AND APPLICATION

Dear God, You are always willing to be my companion and my guide. Thank You for walking with me as I go about the everyday routine of my life. Amen.

Displayed on the signboard of a local church was a succinct message: "Exercise Daily, Walk with the Lord!" This is wise advice for those of us who are serious about becoming all that we can be for God: We are to include God in all the events of our daily Christian walk. As participants in First Place 4 Health, we are asked to include walking in our exercise programs in order to improve our physical health. Take a few minutes now and evaluate how you walk with the Lord on a daily basis:

- Do you "walk in all the way that the LORD your God has commanded you" (Deuteronomy 5:33)?
- Do you "walk before [God] in integrity of heart and uprightness" (1 Kings 9:4)?
- Do you "walk about in freedom" (Psalm 119:45)?
- Do you "walk in the midst of trouble" (Psalm 138:7)?

- Do you "walk in the way of understanding" (Proverbs 9:6)?
- Do you "walk humbly" (Micah 6:8)?
- Have you ever spent time "walking and jumping, and praising God" (Acts 3:8)?
- Do you "walk as Jesus did" (1 John 2:6)?
- Do you "walk in love" (2 John 1:6)?

Being honest about how we walk with God may not be easy, but by being honest, we'll see where we need to improve. The list above may give you some ideas for how to go about making a change or two.

Regardless of the time or circumstances, a walk with Jesus is always an extraordinary event that brings healing, restoration and clarity to those who are willing to allow the risen Lord to be part of their daily stroll through this journey we call life. Each new day is an opportunity to be faithful to our commitment to put God first in our lives and to spend quality time with Him. Walking is not a burden when it is an opportunity to stroll hand in hand with God. Remember always that God is with you as you continue your walk until you reach the ultimate goal!

Dear Lord, Your Word makes clear to me how I should be walking with You. I so want to walk with You as I reach the goal You have waiting for me at the end of my race. Thank You for Your great love for me. Amen.

Group Prayer Requests

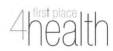

Today's Date: _____

Name	Request

Results

_____

_____

_____

_____

_____

time to
celebrate!

To help shape your brief victory celebration testimony, work through the following questions in your prayer journal:

Day One: List some of the benefits you have gained by allowing the Lord to transform your life through this 12-week First Place 4 Health session. Be sure to list benefits you have received in the physical, mental, emotional and spiritual realms of your being.

Day Two: In what ways have you most significantly changed *mentally*? Have you seen a shift in the ways you think about yourself, food, your relationships or God? How has Scripture memory been a part of these shifts?

Day Three: In what ways have you most significantly changed *emotionally*? Have you begun to identify how your feelings influence your relationship to food and exercise? What are you doing to stay aware of your emotions, both positive and negative?

Day Four: In what ways have you most significantly changed *spiritually*? How has your relationship with God deepened? How has drawing closer to Him made a difference in the other three areas of your life?

Day Five: In what ways have you most significantly changed *physically*? Have you met or exceeded your weight/measurement goals? How has your health improved the past 12 weeks?

Day Six: Was there one person in your First Place 4 Health group who was particularly encouraging to you? How did their kindness make a difference in your First Place 4 Health journey?

Day Seven: Summarize the previous six questions into a one-page testimony, or "faith story," to share at your group's victory celebration.

May our gracious Lord bless and keep you as you continue to keep Him first in all things!

Start Losing, Start Living
leader discussion guide

For in-depth information, guidance and helpful tips about leading a successful First Place 4 Health group, spend time studying the *First Place 4 Health Leader's Guide*. In it, you will find valuable answers to most of your questions, as well as personal insights from many First Place 4 Health group leaders.

For the group meetings in this session, be sure to read and consider each week's discussion topics several days before the meeting—some questions and activities require supplies and/or planning to complete. Also, if you are leading a large group, plan to break into smaller groups for discussion and then come together as a large group to share your answers and responses. Make sure to appoint a capable leader for each small group so that discussions stay focused and on track (and be sure each group records their answers!).

week one: welcome to *Start Losing, Start Living*

During this first week, welcome the members to your group, provide a brief overview of the First Place 4 Health program, explain what is expected of the participants at each of the weekly meetings, and collect the Member Surveys. (See the *First Place 4 Health Leader's Guide* for a detailed outline of how to conduct the first week's meeting.)

week two: receive God's blessing

Invite a volunteer to describe Moses' prayer stance and how important it was to Joshua's success on the battlefield (see Day 1). Go over the importance of prayer partners (like Aaron and Hur). Be sure the group members understand the importance of prayer as they begin this Bible study and their First Place 4 Health journey. Explain that prayers can simply be like conversations with God; they do not have to be something formal, and they certainly do not have to be always the same. Model prayer by beginning and ending each group session with a prayer. And be sure to remind the group members to read the first section in the *First Place 4 Health Member's Guide.*

Go around the group and have each member tell about a symbol or thing that he or she has either used or seen used as a way to remember an event or an instruction (see Day 2). If no one else mentions a cross, point out that many Christians wear a cross as a reminder of what Jesus did for the world.

Discuss the time Joshua and Caleb—along with 10 other men—were sent to scout out the Promised Land (see Day 3). Invite a few volunteers to tell why they think some of the spies doubted God's promise to give the land to His people. Point out that God's Word is filled with stories about how God *did* keep His promises. Make sure the group understands that as we get to know God better and better, we also become more faithful, obeying more easily and better able to be patient and trusting while waiting for God to fulfill all of His promises. If you have time, invite volunteers to tell about a time when one of God's promises held true for them.

Go over the definition of "sanctify" (see Day 4—make holy or godly; make sacred. In other words, the Chosen People were to make themselves clean before God). Part of the way we sanctify ourselves is by making sure that God is a part of every aspect of our lives. Invite volunteers to tell specific things we can do to make sure that God's Word works in us (e.g., memorize memory verses, read the Bible every day, attend a Bible study—like First Place 4 Health).

Invite volunteers to give examples of what freedom will look like for them in regard to their First Place 4 Health endeavors (see Day 5).

Discuss some of the negative messages that people hear from their inner voices that might make people doubt God's promises (see Day 6). Invite volunteers to tell how to stay positive in spite of what an inner voice or the world has to say about anything contrary to God's Word.

Invite a few volunteers to discuss how one of the promises God gave to the Chosen People as they were about to cross the Jordan River relates to them personally (see Day 7).

week three: step out in faith

Begin this week's discussion time by having a member of your group read aloud Joshua 3. After the reading, lead a discussion of what it must have been like for the priests as they stepped into the water, trusting that the waters would part. Remind your group that none of the people crossing the Jordan River that day (with the exception of Joshua and Caleb) had been part of the original group from Egypt who had seen God part the Red Sea. Spend several minutes discussing some of the things God will do when we obey Him and what He will do when we disobey (see Day 1). Remind the group that every one of our actions has a consequence.

Make sure group members understand that we must live in obedience to God's truth, if we expect the Lord to do amazing things for us. In faith we must obediently step forward, trusting that as we do the footwork, God will go before us and provide the results. Of course, we would like for God to part the water before we move forward, but that is not how faith works. Faith is stepping into the rushing water, confident that God will fulfill His promises when we are first willing to obey Him.

Invite volunteers to tell the difference between the old animal sacrifices and the sacrifice Jesus made (see Day 2). Read aloud Hebrews 10:14. Be sure to stress the phrase "has made" so that group members understand that in Christ they have already been made perfect. Make sure, though, that everyone understands we still need to be made holy—cleansed of our sins, because at times we will stumble and fall into sin. Ask volunteers to share how a close relationship with God will help them reach their goals in the First Place 4 Health program and how participation in the program is an opportunity to praise God.

If you have access to a recording of "Joshua Fought the Battle of Jericho," invite your group to sing along with it as it plays (see Day 3). After singing the song, invite a volunteer to relate the entire story of the battle of Jericho. Stress the fact that by following God's instructions—by obeying God—the people were able to make the walls of Jericho come tumbling down.

Point out that we, too, can tear down strongholds by heeding God. Point out that these strongholds are walls that keep us from having a closer walk with God, and then ask for volunteers to describe some of the strongholds that some people need to send tumbling (anger, jealousy, money, beliefs that there are quick fixes to solving weight problems, beliefs that "beautiful people" are the ones we should copy). Discuss how prayer and the Word of God can be used as weapons against the devil's schemes.

Point out to the group that Joshua had lost faith in God because God hadn't "performed" as Joshua had expected when the Chosen People tried to conquer Ai; Joshua questioned God's faithfulness—as we are all prone to do when we have suffered defeat (see Day 4). However, as is always the case, it was not God who had let His people down. Rather, it was the people of Israel who had let God down. Ask volunteers to describe why unconfessed sin is so detrimental not only to us but also to others around us.

Ask for volunteers to explain why without confession there can be no forgiveness of sins (see Day 5). Then ask what shows that our confession is sincere (we turn away from sin and start to do what is right—obeying God; we also start to do good things, good works). Make sure the group members understand that good works by themselves will not mean that the person who performs them will be granted eternal life. Good works by themselves are of no spiritual value. It is faith in Jesus that allows us to have eternal life. It is that faith that then leads us to do good works.

It is also important that group members understand that a believer's sins *do not* separate him or her from God's love. God's love is unconditional and always with us. Even when our hearts grow cold toward God, even when we blatantly disobey Him, His love remains steadfast.

Invite group members to talk about what they learned from reading the stories of some of the people in the Bible (see Days 6 and 7). If you have the time to discuss Rahab's story in some detail, have volunteers tell who Rahab was, what she did, how she is related to Jesus and how her life is a good example of faith in action (see Day 6).

week four: win over deception

Invite a volunteer to explain why circumcision was important for the new generation of the Chosen People (see Day 1—circumcision was a sign that the Chosen People followed God). Make sure group members understand that the new generation of Israelites had to learn about their covenant relationship with God and about their responsibilities to love and serve God wholeheartedly so that they could continue to enjoy God's favor and blessing. Point out that we too must renew our commitment to God, and we need to do that daily. Invite volunteers to tell some of the specific things we should do daily (pray, read the Bible, spend time with like-minded people).

Joshua and the people's taking time to worship God and listen to His commands can be likened to taking time for Sunday worship and/or taking time to attend weekly First Place 4 Health meetings. Remind the group members that keeping God first in all things demands that we take time to do those things that strengthen our relationship with God. Use this as an opportunity to stress the importance of attending group meetings, doing the Bible study every day, memorizing the Scripture verses, and so on.

Invite one of your group members to recount the entire story of the Gibeonite deception (see Day 2). Then lead your group in a discussion about the importance of consulting God rather than relying only on human evidence when making decisions. Invite volunteers to tell some of the ruses to which *we* might fall victim.

Point out to the group that although it is easy to lose heart and become discouraged after we have failed in our responsibility to God, we worship and serve a God of mercy and compassion who forgives our sins and encourages us to continue in our faith (see Day 3). Ask volunteers to tell how they feel about the fact that God has their names written on His palms.

Invite volunteers to tell why we can be so sure that God will indeed fight for us (see Day 4). Ask if anyone in the group has a story that he or she is willing to share either about a time that God fought for him or her in some way or about a time when they were *sure* that God was present and was clearly helping him or her.

Discuss how the words we use can either help or harm someone (see Day 5). Stress the value of encouragement. Invite a volunteer to explain why faith without works is dead. Make sure the group understands that works show that our belief is sincere, that our lives have been transformed and that we obey God's commands. Ask for a volunteer to explain how our words and deeds may influence someone to turn to Christ and start believing in God.

Go over the if-then Scripture exercise with the group (see Day 6). Then invite group members to share their "ifs" and "thens" with the group (see Day 7). Be sure everyone in your group gets a chance to present one of their if-then statements. Remind the group that we only get out of First Place 4 Health what we are willing to put into it. We must do our part before we expect God to abundantly bless us.

week five: build a legacy of faithfulness

Before the group meeting, read Numbers 13 and 14 and Joshua 14, so you will be familiar with the life of Caleb, an amazing man with much to teach us all. Pick one lesson Caleb has for you and share it with your group, and then invite others to share what they have learned from Caleb and how he lived his life.

Discuss how the Spirit we have in us is different from the sort of spirit found in other people (see Day 1). Ask the group about how we should treat the opinions we hear from others.

Ask group members to tell about some of the rewards of being faithful to God (see Day 2). Then ask for some specific ideas about how to avoid evil. Also discuss how steadfast commitment is an important part of the First Place 4 Health program.

Invite volunteers to tell when and how children should be educated about God (see Day 3). Discuss how what we are doing in First Place 4 Health will have positive benefits for our children and grandchildren. Point out that health and fitness practices and traditions can be passed from generation to generation.

Make sure that group members understand that all hope comes from God and that we should never give up hope, just as we should never give up God (see Day 4). Stress the fact that God's love for us is unfailing, and that is enough reason to never give up hope. Ask volunteers to share some specific things we can do so that we "overflow with hope."

On a whiteboard or flip chart, list the fruit of the Spirit as group members tell what gifts they have (see Day 5). Be sure your group understands that the measure of spiritual gifts varies from person to person. Point out that we crucify our sinful natures by giving over to God control of our lives. Then, since we're saved, we're supposed to live as if we have actually done that. Invite someone to explain why we need to cultivate all of the fruit of the Spirit (so it grows bigger in us and so others are attracted to Christ by how they see us talk and behave). If there is time, invite a few volunteers to tell the fruit to which they need to give special attention and how they plan to foster that fruit's growth.

Discuss the fact that without self-control, we will never realize our goals to have balanced lifestyles (see Day 6). Lots of people would like to eliminate self-control from their vocabularies, but point out to the group that we will not bring any of the other parts of the spiritual fruit to maturity without self-control. Go around the group and ask each member to name one benefit they will derive as they exercise a greater degree of self-control.

Lead a discussion about the rhythm of different seasons and how different seasons impact our progress in all aspects of living a balanced lifestyle—emotionally, spiritually, mentally and physically (see Day 7). Consider reading aloud Psalm 1, and emphasize that as we obey God more and more, we will bear more and more fruit, and God will in turn bless us more and more.

week six: draw nearer to God

Discuss the importance of choosing life every day. Stress the fact that choosing life is not a one-time decision, for every day we make individual choices that reinforce (or do not reinforce) our relationship with God. Also talk with your group about how choosing life every day is part of the First Place 4 Health program.

Invite a volunteer to explain why at the same time we are to draw near to God and to resist the devil (see Day 1). Emphasize the fact that to do one without the other is ineffective. Invite volunteers to tell what shows that a person is friendlier with the world than with God (pursues wealth, wants more and more things, chases after beauty according to the world's standards). Be sure to go over the fact that the Holy Spirit is jealous of our love of material things because it means our love is not for God first.

On a whiteboard or flip chart, write the five things we can do to draw nearer to God as described in James 4:7-10 (submit to God, resist the devil, lead a clean or pure life, be sincere about how sad you feel about having sinned, be humble before God). Invite volunteers to tell specific practical things that a person can do to resist the devil and show that he or she serves God (read the Bible, avoid movies [and games] that contain unwholesome content, spend time with other Christians).

Discuss why God helped eliminate the nations in Canaan and why He helps us change "little by little" (see Day 2). Make sure group members understand that as God led His people little by little, little by little they learned to trust Him more and more. God only gave the Israelites as much responsibility as they could handle, and only as they were faithful in little were they given more. In a similar manner, God gives us each challenges that are suited to our spiritual maturity, our circumstances and our relationship to God at the present time. God leads us through a gentle process rather than allowing us to be overwhelmed. God does not take shortcuts, nor does He push us beyond our ability to learn and grow. Giving us one lesson to learn at a time also allows time for us to put the lesson into practice.

Although you may have already discussed the topic of how to grow as a Christian, go over with the group some specific ways to do this (see Day 3). Also invite volunteers to share what they need to leave behind so that they can more easily move ahead.

Invite volunteers to explain why putting on a new self is very much like putting on new clothes (see Day 4). Go over with the group what we should stop doing. Point out that this does not mean, for example, that we can't get angry; what it means is that we should handle anger properly. Emphasize that we are to model the behavior of Jesus (He *did* get angry in the Temple and threw people out of it, but His anger was not malicious; see Matthew 21:12-13).

Discuss what Jesus meant when He said that His followers need to "deny" themselves (see Day 5). Stress that our focus should be on God and what He wants, not on what we want (as Peter did when he rebuked Jesus for predicting His death). Ask someone to explain the difference between what a believer gains by "losing" his or her life as opposed to what a nonbeliever may gain in this life but will ultimately lose (nonbelievers may gain whatever they find pleasing in life, but in the end they lose their souls). Discuss how a person "takes up a cross." Explain to the group that although we are unlikely to literally be nailed to a cross, we do need to be willing to suffer, willing to obey God no matter what problems or troubles we face in our lives.

On a whiteboard or on a flip chart, draw two separate columns. Label one with the heading "I Will Eliminate . . ." and the other column with the heading "I Will Replace It With . . ." (see Day 6). As volunteers give you eliminate/replace-it-with examples, write their answers in the appropriate columns. Stress that while we often give up things that are unique to our situations, some of the things we eliminate are probably common to all of us.

Invite volunteers to share some ideas about what we reveal by how we take care of God's temple, our bodies (see Day 7). Ask the group to apply this to the emotional, spiritual, mental and physical aspects of a balanced lifestyle.

week seven: do your part in the race

Begin your group discussion by talking about how our race to the goal differs from a normal athletic event (see Day 1). Then ask group members to tell how the "great cloud of witnesses" are different from witnesses at a regular athletic event (they not only cheer us on, encouraging us, but they also inspire us by their example).

Invite volunteers to tell how our prize differs from that won in a regular race (see Day 2—our prize is available to *all* runners and it lasts forever). Discuss how we "train" for our race (read the Bible, pray, have discussions with other Christians). Then invite other volunteers to tell specific examples of how other people can "cut in" and cause us to stumble (say things like "One won't hurt," "But this movie won an award, so it's got to be good").

Invite group members to tell why Jesus is such a good example of a runner who finished the race that God set out for Him (see Day 3).

Discuss what went into the creation of each one of us (see Day 4). If you have the time, read aloud Genesis 1:26-31. Note that Psalm 139:13-15 points out that God's character went into each of us at our creation. Invite volunteers to tell how they feel about knowing that God's Spirit is always with them and to tell how that fact affects their behavior.

Point out that the parable of the banquet is really about how people respond to God's invitation to join His kingdom, but the excuses the invited guests give are typical of excuses in general (see Day 5). Ask group members to tell excuses they've heard for people choosing to do something wrong or choosing not to do what they should (it takes too much time; it takes too much energy; everyone else is doing it; no one will notice).

"Not enough time" is a common excuse given to explain why something didn't get done well or completely or didn't get done at all (see Day 6). Talk about time priorities and the importance of weighing all we do in the light of God's priorities, not the priorities of the world. Our responsibility is to arrange our schedules in order to keep God first in all things.

Encourage group members to share whether they are resolute in regard to their goals both in the First Place 4 Health program and in their Christian walk (see Day 7). Invite volunteers to suggest ways that a person can show that he or she is resolute.

Before you close, note for the group that the race we run is more like a marathon than a sprint. We run as long as we live here on earth.

week eight: join with others for success

Invite volunteers to tell the differences between a person who works alone and one who works with others (see Day 1—encouraged, helped in times of trouble/when falter or fall, kept warmer during seasons of cold/despair, able to stand firmer and withstand stormy times). Ask how these advantages are reflected in participation in the First Place 4 Health program.

Point out to the group members that without daily encouragement, all of us are more vulnerable to Satan's schemes, his attempts to outwit us and make us sin (see Day 2). Satan, like a lion, looks particularly for someone who is going through a troubling time, when someone is weak and vulnerable and alone. On a whiteboard or flip chart, write the specific ways group members came up with to encourage others in the group.

Ask a volunteer to tell what the disciples focused on when Jesus told them that they should feed the crowd (see Day 3—the disciples focused on what they didn't have [food and money]). Ask someone to explain what Jesus did before giving out the food and why it was important (Jesus prayed, not for His own benefit, but so the disciples and the crowd would realize from whom the blessing they were about to receive came). Go around the group and invite each group member to tell one blessing they have received by being a participant either in the Bible study or in the First Place 4 Health program.

Discuss the fact that until the teachings of Christ dwell in our hearts, we do not have the internal resources that will allow us to carry out the instructions from our memory verse (see Day 4). Invite someone to tell the definition of "admonish" (to give a gentle warning or sign of disapproval in order to encourage someone to correct a mistake or mend his or her ways). Stress that admonishment is not given in a heavy-handed or harsh manner but given gently, in such a way that a person is actually encouraged by hearing the words of advice. Invite other group members to tell why we should be thankful, even in times of trouble (being thankful reminds us of what we *do* have and allows God to give us peace).

Invite volunteers to tell how the Body of Christ is like a human body (see Days 5 and 7). Make sure the group members understand that because each of us is a different individual, each person serves a different function in the Body and each person is of equal value—each part needs all of the other parts in order to function properly as a whole; like the parts of a human body, we are mutually dependent.

If you have time, invite the group to listen or sing along to a spiritual song of your choice (see Day 6).

week nine: choose whom you will serve

Talk with your group about how God showed His love for us (see Day 1). If anyone in the group had trouble answering the study question about what we should do if we ever become fearful, point out that we can always rely on God's love and the love and support of others during such times. Then ask the group members to explain why loving other Christians is important (shows the world whether we really love God). Invite volunteers to suggest ways that we can sacrifice in order to show love (give our time and/or resources to do something for someone else—run an errand; cook a meal; lend a hand to help build or repair a home; lend a shoulder to cry on or an ear to listen to someone; do an activity someone else wants to do instead of our choice).

Invite volunteers to tell why we should be like Joshua and the Israelites and choose to serve only God (see Day 2). Point out that the repetition of Jewish history reminded the people (as it does for us) of God's provision and goodness, His blessings. On a whiteboard or flip chart, list idols that people worship today as group members tell what they are (money, material things, movie or music stars). Remind group members that removing idols is as important today as it was in Joshua's time, because idols distract us from the One who should be first in our lives.

Discuss with the group some of the things God promises to those who trust in Him (see Day 3). Invite volunteers to share a brief story about a time they relied on their own strength instead of trusting God.

Invite group members to tell why nonbelievers are either foolish or corrupt (see Day 4—fools ignore evidence of God's existence, and wicked people live by their own rules, not God's; they rely on themselves, instead of God). On a whiteboard or flip chart, ask the group members to list ways that we can actively seek God (worship with others, read the Bible, read Bible commentaries, pray).

Lead the group members in a discussion about having to one day account for ourselves in front of God and why or why not that is a scary thought (see Day 5). Invite one volunteer to summarize the parable of the talents, and then ask another volunteer to relate the parable to what we are supposed to do with what God has given each of us.

Before the meeting, read the first two chapters in section 3 of the *First Place 4 Health Member's Guide* to familiarize yourself with accountability and accountability partners (see Day 6). Talk with the group members about the things only a fellow Christian can do for us when we are weak and are having trouble doing what is right emotionally, spiritually, mentally or physically.

Discuss with the group members the importance of having a Paul, a Barnabas and a Timothy in our lives (see Day 7). Invite volunteers to share how they found or were led to the Paul, Barnabas and Timothy in their lives (this might encourage those group members who do not yet have these relationships in their lives).

week ten: recognize God's authority and power

Lead a discussion about what our condition is ("dead" because we are sinful) and what caused us to be able to experience God's resurrection power (see Day 1). Stress that our belief in and close relationship with Jesus makes us able to experience the same power that raised Him from the dead.

Ask the group members to tell over what Jesus has power, and why (see Day 2). Also confirm that all of the group members know what every believer inherits (eternal life guaranteed by the Holy Spirit who lives in every believer). If anyone is unsure about how to answer the question about whom he or she says Jesus is, suggest he or she meet privately with you or a trusted Christian leader to discuss becoming a Christian.

Discuss why Paul wants all believers to know and understand what God wants (see Day 3). Invite volunteers to tell how we learn what God wants us to do (read the Bible, pray, listen for God's voice). Then, with the group members, review what our doing good things does for God (gives Him the glory). On a whiteboard or flip chart, list ways that the world tries to turn us away from our true power source as group members tell what they are (self-help books that urge people to rely solely on their own power in order to make life changes; the assertion that only evolutionary theory is correct; restrictions on where and when "God" can be used in speech). You might also list ways believers can show that they recognize that God is their true power source (say grace in restaurants; treat others kindly, even if they're different from us).

Discuss why Jesus is such a good example for us to follow, especially in regard to His prayer life (see Day 4). Stress that He depended on God as a power source, and He prayed to know His Father's will, for blessing, in thanks. He incorporated prayer not just in the morning or night but throughout the day.

Invite volunteers to tell why we should ask for what we want "in the name of Jesus" (see Day 5). Then ask other volunteers to tell why we don't always get what we ask for (asking in the name of Jesus means asking in/according to God's will; God's will is not always the same as ours, so sometimes God's answer is no, sometimes yes, sometimes not now, sometimes something better; we also must take care not to pray for wrong things or from bad motives).

Invite a volunteer to slowly read aloud Psalm 23 (see Day 6). Then, on a whiteboard or flip chart, make a list as group members share the things our Good Shepherd provides for us.

Discuss in general the sort of people who can lead us to commit a sin or act in a self-destructive way (see Day 7). Then invite volunteers to describe how we should respond when we are asked to participate in or do something we know is wrong in regard to our faith or our First Place 4 Health goals.

week eleven: focus on your ultimate goal

Have the group members talk about the disadvantages of dwelling on the past (see Day 1). Point out that as the Israelites complained about what they used to have in Egypt, they forgot about how cruel the pharaoh and the Egyptians had been. Invite volunteers to briefly describe a time when dwelling on the past hampered their efforts to move forward to reach their First Place 4 Health goals.

Explain to the group that Zephaniah, a prophet and the author of this week's memory verse, was urging the Israelites to turn back to God and rely on Him (see Day 2). God does not delight in arrogant people or on those who depend on their own power or efforts. Invite volunteers to describe how it feels to imagine God rejoicing over them with singing. Then invite other volunteers to tell how we can show our delight in God.

Discuss with the group members how our relationship with God resembles the relationship between a human father and his children (see Day 3). Make sure everyone understands that God's discipline is done for our own good, and it is meted out fairly.

Invite a group member to explain what "fear of the Lord" means (see Day 4). Stress that "fear" in this sense means to revere God, to have a healthy respect for Him and all that He is and has done; it does *not* mean to be scared of God. Go over with the group members examples of "earthly, unspiritual" wisdom (putting self first; thinking that gaining a high status or gaining wealth is most important; "Just do it"; go for whatever you want—such things lead to greed and destruction of self and others). Point out that true wisdom comes from heaven, and then ask for a few specific ideas about how to gain more wisdom.

If possible, show the group members an artist's rendering of what the New Jerusalem might look like (see Day 5). Invite three different group members to tell what Jesus told us about heaven (such as He is preparing a place for us, He will come back for us, and we know the way to get there).

Consider making copies of a maze for each group member to complete (see Day 6). Discuss with group members how each of our lives is much more like a maze than a straight line. Invite volunteers to share where they are on their journeys and what they plan to do next.

Discuss how walking with God helps us attain both the ultimate goal we seek as well as one of our goals for First Place 4 Health (see Day 7). Invite volunteers to share their evaluation of how they walk with God and where they are on their walk with God.

week twelve: time to celebrate!

Even though most of your meeting this week will be a victory celebration, take some time at the beginning of the meeting to talk about how much God loves each person in the group and how each of us is called to love our brothers and sisters in Christ. (See "Planning a Victory Celebration" in the First Place 4 Health Leader's Guide for ideas about throwing a successful celebration for your group.)

For the rest of the study time, allow each member to tell his or her Start Losing, Start Living story. Give members an equal opportunity to share the goals they set for themselves at the beginning of the session and talk about the challenges and good things God has done for them throughout the process. Don't allow the more talkative group members to monopolize the conversation. Even the quiet members need an opportunity to share their stories and successes! Even those who have not met their goals have still been part of the journey, so allow them to share and talk about why they did not succeed.

Making a commitment to continue in First Place 4 Health is an important part of victory. Be sure to talk about your group's future plans, and make each person feel welcome to continue to journey with you.

Close your Victory Celebration by blessing the members of your group with the words the priests in Joshua's day would have used to bless God's Chosen People:

"The LORD bless you and keep you; the LORD make his face shine upon you and be gracious to you; the LORD turn his face toward you and give you peace" (Numbers 6:24-26).

First Place 4 Health menu plans

Each menu plan is based on approximately 1,400 to 1,500 calories per day. All recipe and menu exchanges were determined using the Master-Cook software, a program that accesses a database containing more than 6,000 food items prepared using the United States Department of Agriculture (USDA) publications and information from food manufacturers. As with any nutritional program, MasterCook calculates the nutritional values of the recipes based on ingredients. Nutrition may vary due to how the food is prepared, where the food comes from, soil content, season, ripeness, processing and method of preparation. For these reasons, please use the recipes and menu plans as approximate guides. Consult a physician and/or a registered dietitian before starting a weight-loss program.

For those who need more calories, add the following to the 1,400-calorie plan:

- 1,800 calories: 2 ounce equivalent of meat, 3 ounce equivalent of bread, ½ cup vegetable serving, 1 tsp. fat

- 2,000 calories: 2 ounce equivalent of meat, 4 ounce equivalent of bread, ½ cup vegetable serving, 3 tsp. fat

- 2,200 calories: 2 ounce equivalent of meat, 5 ounce equivalent of bread, ½ cup vegetable serving, ½ cup fruit serving, 5 tsp. fat

- 2,400 calories: 2 ounce equivalent of meat, 6 ounce equivalent of bread, 1 cup vegetable serving, ½ cup fruit serving, 6 tsp. fat

First Week Grocery List

Produce
- [ ] arugula, baby
- [ ] asparagus
- [ ] avocado
- [ ] bananas
- [ ] basil
- [ ] bean sprouts
- [ ] beefsteak tomato
- [ ] Boston lettuce leaves
- [ ] broccoli
- [ ] cantaloupe
- [ ] carrots
- [ ] cherry tomatoes
- [ ] chives
- [ ] cucumber
- [ ] Gala apples
- [ ] garlic cloves
- [ ] ginger
- [ ] Granny Smith apple
- [ ] green onions
- [ ] green Thai chile
- [ ] jicama
- [ ] leek
- [ ] lemons
- [ ] mint leaves
- [ ] onions
- [ ] oregano
- [ ] parsley, flat-leaf
- [ ] radishes
- [ ] raisins
- [ ] red bell peppers
- [ ] red onions
- [ ] red pepper
- [ ] red potatoes
- [ ] Savoy cabbage
- [ ] shallots
- [ ] snow peas
- [ ] spinach, baby
- [ ] sugar snap peas
- [ ] sweet mini peppers
- [ ] thyme leaves
- [ ] tomatoes
- [ ] turnip
- [ ] yellow squash
- [ ] zucchini

Baking/Cooking Products
- [ ] almond paste
- [ ] baking powder
- [ ] baking spray with flour (such as Baker's Joy®)
- [ ] canola oil
- [ ] cornstarch
- [ ] dark brown sugar
- [ ] flour, all-purpose
- [ ] nonstick cooking spray
- [ ] olive oil, extra-virgin
- [ ] panko (Japanese breadcrumbs)
- [ ] peanut oil
- [ ] powdered sugar
- [ ] sesame oil, dark
- [ ] sugar
- [ ] vanilla extract
- [ ] white wine, dry

Spices
- [ ] bay leaf
- [ ] black pepper
- [ ] cinnamon
- [ ] herbes de Provence
- [ ] nutmeg
- [ ] paprika
- [ ] salt

Nuts/Seeds
- [ ] almonds
- [ ] cashews, unsalted
- [ ] pine nuts

Condiments, Spreads and Sauces
- [ ] cider vinegar
- [ ] Dijon mustard
- [ ] hoisin sauce
- [ ] honey
- [ ] ketchup
- [ ] pesto
- [ ] rice vinegar
- [ ] soy sauce, lower-sodium
- [ ] white wine vinegar

Breads, Cereals and Pasta
- [ ] bread, multigrain
- [ ] bread, whole-wheat
- [ ] country bread
- [ ] French bread
- [ ] Grape Nuts®
- [ ] oatmeal
- [ ] penne (pasta)
- [ ] puffed rice cereal
- [ ] quinoa
- [ ] rice noodles (pad thai noodles)
- [ ] rice, long-grain boil-in-bag

Canned/Frozen Foods
- [ ] cannellini beans or other white beans
- [ ] chicken broth, fat-free, lower-sodium
- [ ] chile paste
- [ ] cremini mushrooms, pre-sliced
- [ ] pearl onions
- [ ] pie dough
- [ ] pizza dough
- [ ] red pepper hummus
- [ ] tomatoes, no-salt-added

Dairy Products
- [ ] butter
- [ ] Greek yogurt, 2% reduced-fat, plain
- [ ] Gruyère cheese
- [ ] margarine, light
- [ ] milk, 1% lowfat
- [ ] milk, nonfat
- [ ] mozzarella cheese, part-skim
- [ ] Parmesan cheese
- [ ] Parmigiano-Reggiano cheese
- [ ] pecorino Romano cheese
- [ ] queso fresco
- [ ] Swiss cheese
- [ ] yogurt, fat-free

Juices
- [ ] lemon juice
- [ ] lime juice

Meat and Poultry
- [ ] chicken breast halves, skinless and boneless
- [ ] eggs
- [ ] ham hock, smoked
- [ ] lamb, lean-ground
- [ ] pancetta
- [ ] pork loin chops, bone-in center-cut
- [ ] salmon fillets (such as wild Alaskan)
- [ ] shrimp
- [ ] sirloin steak, boneless
- [ ] turkey breast, deli-style

First Week Meals and Recipes

DAY 1

Breakfast

Fried Egg and Mushroom Sandwich

4 tsp. extra-virgin olive oil, divided
1 cup shallots, thinly sliced
  and divided
1 (8-oz.) package cremini
  mushrooms, pre-sliced
2 tbsp. dry white wine
½ tsp. black pepper, divided
¼ tsp. salt

8 tsp. pesto, refrigerated
4 (1½-oz.) slices multigrain
  bread
2 oz. Parmigiano-Reggiano cheese
  (about ½ cup), grated
4 large eggs
8 (¼-inch-thick) slices tomato
3 tbsp. fresh basil, chopped

Heat a large nonstick skillet over medium heat. Add 2 teaspoons oil to pan; swirl to coat. Add ⅔ cup shallots; cook 3 minutes. Add mushrooms; cook 4 minutes or until tender, stirring occasionally. Add wine, ¼ teaspoon pepper and salt; bring to a boil, scraping pan to loosen browned bits. Cook 2 minutes or until liquid almost evaporates, stirring occasionally. Remove mushroom mixture from pan; keep warm. Return pan to medium heat. Add 1 teaspoon oil to pan; swirl to coat. Add remaining ⅓ cup shallots. Sauté 5 minutes or until lightly browned. Remove shallots from pan; keep warm. Preheat broiler to high. Spread 2 teaspoons pesto over one side of each bread slice. Top each slice with about 2 tablespoons cheese. Broil 2 minutes or until cheese melts; keep warm. Return pan to medium heat. Add remaining 1 teaspoon oil to pan; swirl to coat. Crack eggs into pan and cook 4 minutes or until whites are set. Top each bread slice with 2 tomato slices. Divide mushroom mixture evenly among bread slices and top each serving with 1 egg. Sprinkle with remaining ¼ teaspoon pepper, shallots and basil. Serves 4.

Nutritional Information: 378 calories; 19g fat; 20g protein; 32g carbohydrate; 5g dietary fiber; 32mg cholesterol; 623mg sodium.

Lunch

Sugar Snap Slaw and BBQ Salmon

2 tbsp. dark sesame oil, divided
3 garlic cloves, crushed

1 (½-inch) fresh ginger, peeled
2 tbsp. lime juice

2 tbsp. lower-sodium soy sauce
1½ tbsp. ketchup
2 tsp. dark brown sugar
1 tsp. chile paste, ground
¼ tsp. salt
4 (6-oz.) frozen salmon fillets (such as wild Alaskan), thawed

2 cups sugar snap peas, trimmed and thinly sliced crosswise
½ cup radishes, grated
¼ cup shallots, thinly vertically sliced
2 tsp. rice vinegar
nonstick cooking spray

Preheat the grill to high heat. Combine 1 tablespoon oil, garlic and ginger in a mini food processor; pulse until finely chopped. Add lime juice, soy sauce, ketchup, brown sugar and chile paste; pulse to combine. Place salmon on a grill rack coated with nonstick cooking spray; brush tops of salmon with half of sauce. Grill 10 minutes; brush with remaining sauce. Grill an additional 10 minutes or until desired degree of doneness. Combine peas, radishes and shallots. Combine vinegar and remaining 1 tablespoon oil, stirring well; drizzle over pea mixture. Sprinkle with salt and toss. Serve with salmon. Serves 4 (1 fillet and ¾ cup slaw).

Nutritional Information: 268 calories; 11g fat; 28g protein; 13g carbohydrate; 2g dietary fiber; 66mg cholesterol; 474mg sodium.

Dinner

Pork Chops Topped with Apples and Onions

2½ tsp. canola oil, divided
1½ cups frozen pearl onions, thawed
2 cups Gala apple wedges
1 tbsp. butter, divided
2 tsp. fresh thyme leaves
½ tsp. salt, divided
½ tsp. black pepper, divided

4 (6-oz.) bone-in center-cut pork loin chops (about ½-inch thick)
½ cup fat-free, lower-sodium chicken broth
½ tsp. all-purpose flour
1 tsp. cider vinegar

Preheat oven to 400° F. Heat a large ovenproof skillet over medium-high heat. Add 1 teaspoon oil to pan; swirl to coat. Pat onions dry with a paper towel. Add onions to pan; cook 2 minutes or until lightly browned, stirring once. Add apples to pan; place in oven. Bake at 400° F or 10 minutes or until onions and apple are tender. Stir in 2 teaspoons butter, thyme, ¼ teaspoon salt and ¼ teaspoon pepper. Heat a large skillet over medium-high heat. Sprinkle pork with remaining ¼ teaspoon salt and ¼ teaspoon pepper. Add remaining 1½ teaspoons oil to pan; swirl to coat. Add pork to pan; cook 3 minutes on each side or until desired degree of doneness. Remove pork from pan; keep warm. Combine broth and flour in a small bowl, stirring with a whisk. Add broth mixture to pan; bring to a boil, scraping pan to loosen browned bits. Cook 1 minute or until reduced to ¼ cup. Stir in vinegar and remaining 1 teaspoon butter. Serve sauce with pork and apple mixture. Serves 4.

Nutritional Information: 240 calories; 10g fat; 25g protein; 11g carbohydrate; 2g dietary fiber; 84mg cholesterol; 379mg sodium.

DAY 2

Breakfast

Almond Bread

1½ cups all-purpose flour	½ tsp. vanilla extract
1½ tsp. baking powder	½ cup plus 1 tbsp. nonfat milk,
½ tsp. salt	divided
⅔ cup sugar	baking spray with flour
2 tbsp. butter, softened	(such as Baker's Joy®)
2 tbsp. canola oil	¼ cup almonds, sliced
1 (7-oz.) package almond paste	⅓ cup powdered sugar
2 large eggs	dash of salt

Preheat oven to 350° F. Lightly spoon flour into dry measuring cups; level with a knife. Combine flour, baking powder and salt, stirring well with a whisk. Place granulated sugar, butter and almond paste in a large bowl; beat with a mixer at medium speed until well combined (about 3 minutes). Add eggs, 1 at a time, beating well after each addition; beat in vanilla. Beating at low speed, add flour mixture and ½ cup milk alternately to butter mixture, beginning and ending with flour mixture; beat just until combined. Scrape batter into a 9" x 5" metal loaf pan coated with baking spray; sprinkle with sliced almonds. Bake at 350° F for 50 minutes or until a wooden pick inserted in the center comes out with moist crumbs clinging. Cool in pan on a wire rack 10 minutes. Remove from pan; cool on wire rack. Place powdered sugar in a small bowl. Add remaining 1 tablespoon milk and dash of salt; stir with a whisk until smooth. Drizzle glaze over top of bread; let stand until set. Serves 16.

Nutritional Information: 190 calories; 6g fat; 4g protein; 27g carbohydrate; 1g dietary fiber; 27mg cholesterol; 144mg sodium.

Lunch

Grilled Lemon Shrimp Salad

2 tsp. lemon rind, grated
½ tsp. paprika
½ tsp. salt, divided
½ tsp. black pepper, divided
7 tsp. extra-virgin olive oil, divided
24 extra-large shrimp, peeled and
   deveined (about 1 lb.)
6 cups baby arugula
1 avocado, peeled and diced

1 cup jicama, peeled and cut into
   2″ x ¼″ strips
2 tbsp. lemon juice
1 tbsp. white wine vinegar
¼ tsp. sugar
1 oz. queso fresco (about ¼ cup),
   crumbled
nonstick cooking spray

Preheat grill to high heat. Combine rind, paprika, ¼ teaspoon salt, ¼ teaspoon pepper, 1 teaspoon oil and shrimp in a medium bowl. Thread 4 shrimp onto each of 6 (10-inch) skewers. Coat grill rack with nonstick cooking spray. Grill shrimp 2 minutes on each side or until done. Remove shrimp from skewers. Combine shrimp, arugula, jicama and avocado in a large bowl; toss gently. Combine remaining 2 tablespoons oil, remaining ¼ teaspoon salt, remaining ¼ teaspoon pepper, lemon juice, vinegar and sugar in a small bowl, stirring with a whisk. Add juice mixture to shrimp mixture and toss gently to coat. Divide the salad among 4 large plates; sprinkle evenly with queso fresco. Serves 4.

Nutritional Information: 309 calories; 18g fat; 26g protein; 11g carbohydrate; 6g dietary fiber; 175mg cholesterol; 430mg sodium.

Dinner

Tomato Asparagus Carbonara

3 quarts water
1 tbsp. extra-virgin olive oil
1 lb. (1-inch) asparagus, trimmed
   and diagonally cut
3 garlic cloves, minced
1 pint cherry tomatoes, halved
½ tsp. salt

½ tsp. black pepper
2 oz. pecorino Romano cheese
   (about ½ cup), finely grated
1 large egg
8 oz. penne pasta, uncooked
¼ cup fresh basil

Bring 3 quarts water to a boil in a Dutch oven. Heat a large nonstick skillet over medium-high heat. Add oil to pan; swirl to coat. Add asparagus; sauté 3½ minutes. Add garlic; sauté for 1 minute. Add tomatoes; cook for

6 minutes or until tomatoes are tender. Combine cheese, salt, pepper and egg in a large bowl, stirring with a whisk. Add pasta to boiling water; cook 10 minutes or until al dente. Drain and toss pasta immediately with egg mixture. Add tomato mixture, tossing until sauce thickens. Divide pasta equally among 4 bowls. Sprinkle each serving with 1 tablespoon basil. Serve immediately. Serves 4.

Nutritional Information: 335 calories; 9g fat; 15g protein; 51g carbohydrate; 5g dietary fiber; 63mg cholesterol; 447mg sodium.

DAY 3

Breakfast
1 cup puffed rice cereal   ½ banana, sliced
1 cup nonfat milk

Nutritional Information: 194 calories; 1g fat; 10g protein; 38g carbohydrate; 2g dietary fiber; 4mg cholesterol; 127mg sodium.

Lunch

Lettuce Wraps with Spiced Lamb

2 tsp. canola oil   ½ cup tomato, chopped
1 cup onion, finely chopped   ½ cup cucumber, chopped
2 tsp. garlic cloves, minced   ¼ cup plain 2% reduced-fat
1 tsp. cinnamon   Greek yogurt
¾ tsp. salt   ¼ cup red pepper hummus
¼ tsp. black pepper   8 Boston lettuce leaves
6 oz. lean-ground lamb   2 tbsp. mint leaves, torn
½ cup fresh flat-leaf parsley, chopped   1 tbsp. pine nuts, toasted

Heat a large skillet over high heat. Add oil to pan; swirl to coat. Add onion, garlic, cinnamon, salt and lamb to pan; sauté 5 minutes or until lamb is done. Combine parsley, tomato and cucumber in a medium bowl. Stir in lamb mixture. Combine yogurt and hummus in a small bowl. Place about ¼ cup lamb mixture in each lettuce leaf. Top each wrap with 1 tablespoon hummus mixture. Divide mint and pine nuts evenly among wraps. Serves 4 (2 wraps each).

Nutritional Information: 158 calories; 8g fat; 11g protein; 11g carbohydrate; 3g dietary fiber; 24mg cholesterol; 488mg sodium.

Dinner

Chicken Cordon Bleu

4 (6-oz.) skinless, boneless chicken breast halves	1 large egg
½ tsp. black pepper	2½ oz. Gruyère cheese (about 10 tbsp.), shredded and divided
¼ tsp. salt	1 tbsp. fresh thyme leaves, chopped
¾ cup panko (Japanese breadcrumbs)	2 garlic cloves, minced
½ cup all-purpose flour	4 slices pancetta (about 1¼ oz.)
1 tbsp. water	nonstick cooking spray

Preheat oven to 350° F. Place chicken between 2 sheets of plastic wrap; pound to ¼-inch thickness. Sprinkle chicken evenly with pepper and salt. Heat a skillet over medium heat. Add panko; cook 2 minutes or until toasted, stirring often. Remove from heat. Place flour in a dish. Combine 1 tablespoon water and egg in a bowl; lightly beat. Pour egg mixture into a dish. Combine panko, 2 tablespoons cheese, thyme and garlic in a dish. Working with 1 piece of chicken at a time, dredge in flour. Dip in egg mixture; dredge in panko mixture. Top with 1 pancetta slice and 2 tablespoons cheese. Roll up; secure with a toothpick. Place roll, seam side down, on a wire rack coated with nonstick cooking spray. Place rack on a baking sheet. Repeat procedure with remaining ingredients. Bake at 350° F for 25 minutes or until chicken is done. Serves 4.

Nutritional Information: 414 calories; 12g fat; 51g protein; 21g carbohydrate; 1g dietary fiber; 169mg cholesterol; 513mg sodium.

DAY 4

Breakfast

Quiche Muffins

1 tbsp. extra-virgin olive oil	¼ cup 1% lowfat milk
¼ cup onion, diced	½ tsp. salt
1 cup baby spinach, coarsely chopped	¼ tsp. black pepper
	4 large eggs
2 oz. part-skim mozzarella cheese (about ½ cup), shredded	nonstick cooking spray

Preheat oven to 350° F. Coat 6 muffin cups with nonstick cooking spray. Heat a medium nonstick skillet over medium-high heat. Add oil; swirl to coat. Add onion; sauté 3 minutes or until almost tender. Add spinach; sauté 2 minutes or just until spinach begins to wilt, stirring constantly. Transfer spinach mixture to a small bowl; cool 3 minutes. Stir in cheese. Combine milk, salt, pepper and eggs, stirring with a whisk until blended. Stir in cheese mixture. Divide mixture evenly among prepared muffin cups. Bake at 350° F for 20 minutes or until puffed and set. (Quiches will deflate slightly as they cool.) Serve warm. Serves 6.

Nutritional Information: 108 calories; 8g fat; 7g protein; 2g carbohydrate; trace dietary fiber; 147mg cholesterol; 268mg sodium.

Lunch

Vegetable Ham Stew

4 oz. dried cannellini or
  Great Northern beans
1 tbsp. extra-virgin olive oil
1 cup onion, chopped
1½ cups leek, thinly sliced
4 garlic cloves, chopped
4 cups chicken broth, fat-free, lower-
  sodium
½ tsp. herbes de Provence, dried
1 smoked ham hock (about 8 oz.),
  cross-cut
1 bay leaf

6 oz. red potatoes, cubed
6 oz. turnip, cubed
1 large carrot, cubed
4 cups Savoy cabbage, thinly sliced
¼ cup fresh flat-leaf parsley, chopped
2 tbsp. fresh thyme leaves, chopped
1½ tbsp. cider vinegar
½ tsp. salt
½ tsp. black pepper
6 (1-oz.) slices country bread, toasted
1 garlic clove, halved
1 tbsp. butter, softened

Sort and wash beans. Place in a large Dutch oven. Cover with water to 2 inches above beans. Cover and let stand for 8 hours or overnight. Drain. Heat oil in a large Dutch oven over medium heat; swirl to coat. Add onion. Cover and cook 8 minutes or until tender, stirring occasionally. Add leek and chopped garlic; cook 2 minutes, stirring occasionally. Add soaked beans, stock, herbes de Provence, ham hocks and bay leaf. Bring to a boil. Cover, reduce heat and simmer 1 hour or until beans are just tender. Remove ham hock; cool slightly. Pick meat from bones; reserve meat. Discard bones and fat. Add potatoes, turnip and carrot to pan; cook 10 minutes or until tender. Stir in cabbage; simmer 4 minutes. Stir in parsley, thyme, vinegar, salt and black pepper. Rub toast slices with cut sides of garlic clove; spread evenly with butter. Serve toast with soup. Serves 6.

Nutritional Information: 235 calories; 7g fat; 13g protein; 31g carbohydrate; 7g dietary fiber; 28mg cholesterol; 645mg sodium.

Dinner

Fresh Spinach and Onion Pizza

12 oz. refrigerated fresh pizza dough
1 tbsp. canola oil, divided
2 cups onion (about ½ large),
    vertically sliced
6 garlic cloves, thinly sliced
1 (28½-oz.) can no-salt-added
    tomatoes, chopped
¾ tsp. crushed red pepper

2 tbsp. fresh oregano, chopped
    and divided
¼ tsp. salt
3 oz. part-skim mozzarella cheese,
    torn into bite-sized pieces
1½ oz. Parmesan cheese, grated
    (about ⅓ cup)
4 oz. fresh baby spinach

Remove dough from refrigerator. Let stand at room temperature, covered, 30 minutes. Place a heavy baking sheet in oven. Preheat oven to 500° F (keep baking sheet in oven as it preheats). Heat a large nonstick skillet over medium heat. Add 1 teaspoon oil to pan; swirl to coat. Add onion; cook 4 minutes or until softened, stirring frequently. Remove onion from pan. Add 1 teaspoon oil to pan; swirl to coat. Add garlic; cook 1 minute, stirring frequently. Add tomatoes, 1 tablespoon oregano, pepper and salt; cook 4 minutes or until most of liquid evaporates, stirring mixture occasionally. Roll dough into a 13-inch circle on a lightly floured surface; pierce entire surface liberally with a fork. Carefully place dough on preheated baking sheet. Spread tomato mixture evenly over dough, leaving a ½-inch border. Top with onion and cheeses. Bake at 500° F for 12 minutes or until crust is golden and cheese is lightly browned. Heat a large nonstick skillet over medium-high heat. Add remaining 1 teaspoon oil to pan; swirl to coat. Add spinach; sauté 2 minutes or until spinach wilts. Top pizza with remaining 1 tablespoon oregano and spinach. Cut into 8 slices. Serves 4.

Nutritional Information: 407 calories; 13g fat; 18g protein; 54g carbohydrate; 9g dietary fiber; 27mg cholesterol; 716mg sodium.

DAY 5

Breakfast

⅓ medium cantaloupe
1 cup fat-free yogurt

¼ cup Grape Nuts® cereal (sprinkled
    over yogurt)

Nutritional Information: 281 calories; 1g fat; 15g protein; 57g carbohydrate; 5g dietary fiber; 3mg cholesterol; 345mg sodium.

Lunch

White Bean Salad with Herbed Shrimp

1 red bell pepper
4 cups baby arugula, loosely packed
½ cup red onion, thinly
   vertically sliced
2 tbsp. fresh chives, chopped
2 tbsp. fresh basil, chopped
1 tbsp. fresh flat-leaf parsley,
   chopped
1 (15-oz.) can cannellini beans or
   Great Northern beans, rinsed
   and drained

½ tsp. lemon rind, grated
2 tbsp. lemon juice
1 garlic clove, minced
3 tbsp. extra-virgin olive oil
¼ tsp. salt, divided
¼ tsp. black pepper, divided
1 lb. large shrimp, peeled
   and deveined
2 tbsp. pine nuts, toasted
nonstick cooking spray

Preheat broiler to high. Halve bell pepper lengthwise; discard seeds and membranes. Place halves, skin sides up, on a baking sheet. Broil 12 minutes or until blackened. Seal in a paper bag. Let stand 5 minutes. Peel and chop. Combine bell pepper, arugula, red onion, chives, basil, parsley and white beans. In separate small bowl, combine rind, juice, garlic, oil, ⅛ teaspoon salt and ⅛ teaspoon pepper. Heat a large skillet over medium-high heat. Coat pan with nonstick cooking spray. Sprinkle shrimp with remaining salt and pepper. Cook 2 minutes on each side or until done. Add shrimp, lemon mixture and nuts to arugula mixture; toss. Serves 4.

Nutritional Information: 326 calories; 16g fat; 29g protein; 17g carbohydrate; 5g dietary fiber; 172mg cholesterol; 494mg sodium.

Dinner

Squash, Tomato and Red Pepper Gratin

5 tsp. extra virgin olive oil, divided
2 cups red onion, chopped
1½ cups red bell pepper, chopped
1 lb. yellow squash, cut into ¼"-thick
   slices (about 3½ cups)
1 tbsp. garlic cloves, minced
½ cup cooked quinoa
½ cup fresh basil, thinly sliced
   and divided
1½ tsp. fresh thyme leaves, chopped

¾ tsp. salt, divided
½ tsp. black pepper
½ cup nonfat milk
3 oz. aged Gruyère cheese, shredded
   (about ¾ cup)
3 large eggs, lightly beaten
1½ oz. French bread baguette, torn
1 (12-oz.) beefsteak tomato, seeded
   and cut into 8 slices
nonstick cooking spray

Preheat oven to 375° F. Heat a large nonstick skillet over medium heat. Add 4 teaspoons oil; swirl to coat. Add onion; cook 3 minutes. Add bell pepper; cook 2 minutes. Add squash and garlic; cook 4 minutes. Place vegetable mixture in a large bowl. Stir in quinoa, ¼ cup basil, thyme, ½ teaspoon salt and black pepper. Combine remaining ¼ teaspoon salt, milk, cheese and eggs in a medium bowl, stirring with a whisk. Add milk mixture to vegetable mixture, stirring until just combined. Spoon mixture into an 11" x 7" glass or ceramic baking dish coated with nonstick cooking spray. Place bread in a food processor; pulse until coarse crumbs form. Return skillet to medium-high heat. Add remaining 1 teaspoon oil to pan; swirl to coat. Add breadcrumbs; cook 3 minutes or until toasted. Arrange tomatoes evenly over vegetable mixture. Top evenly with breadcrumbs. Bake at 375° F for 40 minutes or until topping is browned. Sprinkle with remaining ¼ cup basil. Serves 6.

Nutritional Information: 235 calories; 12g fat; 12g protein; 21g carbohydrate; 4g dietary fiber; 123mg cholesterol; 443mg sodium.

DAY 6

Breakfast

1 cup oatmeal with ¼ tsp. light margarine, dash nutmeg, dash cinnamon, 1 cup nonfat milk and 2 tbsp. raisins

Nutritional Information: 284 calories; 3g fat; 15g protein; 50g carbohydrate; 5g dietary fiber; 4mg cholesterol; 517mg sodium.

Lunch

Zucchini and Onion Quiche

½ (14.1-oz.) package refrigerated pie dough
1 tbsp. extra-virgin olive oil
4 cups (⅛-inch-thick) slices zucchini
3 garlic cloves, minced
¾ tsp. salt, divided
1 cup nonfat milk

½ cup caramelized onions, finely chopped
1½ tbsp. all-purpose flour
½ tsp. black pepper
3 large eggs
2 oz. Parmigiano-Reggiano cheese, grated (about ½ cup)

Preheat oven to 425° F. Roll dough into a 12-inch circle. Fit dough into a 10" deep-dish pie plate. Fold edges under and flute. Line dough with foil;

arrange pie weights or dried beans on foil. Bake at 425° F for 12 minutes or until edges are golden. Remove weights and foil; bake an additional 2 minutes. Cool on a wire rack. Reduce oven temperature to 375° F. Heat a large non-stick skillet over medium-high heat. Add oil to pan; swirl. Add zucchini and garlic; sprinkle with ¼ teaspoon salt. Sauté 5 minutes or until crisp-tender. Cool slightly. Arrange caramelized onions over bottom of crust; top with zucchini mixture. Combine remaining ½ teaspoon salt, milk, flour, pepper, eggs and cheese in a medium bowl, stirring well with a whisk. Pour milk mixture over zucchini mixture. Bake at 375° F for 35 minutes or until set. Let stand 10 minutes before serving. Serves 6.

Nutritional Information: 314 calories; 18g fat; 10g protein; 29g carbohydrate; 2g dietary fiber; 119mg cholesterol; 564mg sodium.

....

Dinner

Sweet and Spicy Shrimp with Rice Noodles

1 tbsp. rice vinegar	2 tbsp. unsalted cashews, chopped
2½ tsp. honey	2 tsp. fresh ginger, peeled and
1 tbsp. chile paste, ground	chopped
1 tbsp. lower-sodium soy sauce	1 green Thai chile, halved
12 oz. medium shrimp, peeled	12 sweet mini peppers, halved
and deveined	¾ cup carrot, matchstick-cut
4 oz. flat rice noodles, uncooked	¼ tsp. salt
1 tbsp. peanut oil	¾ cup snow peas, trimmed
1 tbsp. garlic cloves, thinly sliced	¾ cup fresh bean sprouts

Combine rice vinegar, honey, chile paste and soy sauce in a medium bowl, stirring well with a whisk. Add shrimp to vinegar mixture; toss to coat. Cover and refrigerate 30 minutes. Cook noodles according to package directions, omitting salt and fat; drain. Rinse with cold water; drain. Heat a large skillet or wok over medium-high heat. Add oil to pan; swirl to coat. Add cashews, garlic, ginger, and Thai chile to pan; stir-fry 1 minute or until garlic begins to brown. Remove cashew mixture from pan with a slotted spoon and set aside. Increase heat to high. Add sweet peppers, carrot and salt to pan; stir-fry 2 minutes. Add shrimp mixture (do not drain); stir-fry 2 minutes. Stir in noodles and peas; cook 1 minute, tossing to coat. Return cashew mixture to pan. Add bean sprouts; cook 1 minute or until thoroughly heated, tossing frequently. Serves 4.

Nutritional Information: 299 calories; 9g fat; 22g protein; 34g carbohydrate; 3g dietary fiber; 129mg cholesterol; 492mg sodium.

DAY 7

Breakfast

Banana Smoothie

½ cup 1% lowfat milk
½ cup ice, crushed
1 tbsp. honey
⅛ tsp. ground nutmeg

1 frozen large banana, sliced
1 cup plain 2% reduced-fat
  Greek yogurt

Combine milk, ice, honey, nutmeg and banana in a blender; process 2 minutes or until smooth. Add yogurt; process just until blended. Serve immediately. Serves 2.

Nutritional Information: 212 calories; 4g fat; 14g protein; 34g carbohydrate; 2g dietary fiber; 9mg cholesterol; 75mg sodium.

Lunch

Turkey, Apple and Swiss Melt

1 tbsp. Dijon mustard
8 (1-oz.) slices whole-wheat bread
4 (1-oz.) slices Swiss cheese
1 small (5-oz.) Granny Smith apple,
  thinly sliced

1 tbsp. honey
8 oz. lower-sodium deli turkey
  breast, thinly sliced
nonstick cooking spray

Combine mustard and honey in a small bowl. Spread one side of each of 4 bread slices with 1½ teaspoons mustard mixture. Place one cheese slice on dressed side of bread slices; top each with 5 apple slices and 2 ounces turkey. Top sandwiches with remaining 4 bread slices. Coat both sides of sandwiches with nonstick cooking spray. Heat a large nonstick skillet over medium-high heat. Add sandwiches to pan. Cook 2 minutes on each side or until bread is browned and cheese melts. Serves 4.

Nutritional Information: 350 calories; 11g fat; 27g protein; 35g carbohydrate; 4g dietary fiber; 46mg cholesterol; 758mg sodium.

Dinner

Beef and Broccoli over Rice

1 (3½-oz.) bag boil-in-bag long-
  grain rice

¼ cup lower-sodium soy sauce
1 tbsp. cornstarch

1 tbsp. hoisin sauce

1 (12-oz.) boneless sirloin steak, cut into thin strips

2 tsp. canola oil

2 cups broccoli florets

1 cup red onion, vertically sliced

1 cup carrot, chopped

½ cup water

2 tsp. dark sesame oil

⅓ cup green onions, sliced

Cook rice according to the package directions. Combine soy sauce, cornstarch and hoisin in a medium bowl. Add beef; toss to coat. Heat a large skillet over high heat. Add oil to pan; swirl to coat. Remove beef, reserving marinade. Add beef to pan; cook 2 minutes or until browned, stirring occasionally. Remove beef from pan. Add broccoli and next 4 ingredients (through sesame oil) to pan; cook 4 minutes or until broccoli is crisp-tender, stirring occasionally. Add reserved marinade to pan; bring to a boil. Cook 1 minute. Add beef to pan; cook 1 minute or until thoroughly heated. Sprinkle with green onions. Serve over rice. Serves 4.

Nutritional Information: 311 calories; 9g fat; 24g protein; 32g carbohydrate; 3g dietary fiber; 36mg cholesterol; 529mg sodium.

Second Week Grocery List

Produce

- ❏ arugula or watercress
- ❏ baby bok choy
- ❏ baking potato
- ❏ bananas
- ❏ basil
- ❏ blackberries
- ❏ blueberries
- ❏ Boston lettuce leaves
- ❏ carrots
- ❏ cauliflower
- ❏ cherries
- ❏ cherry tomatoes, multicolored
- ❏ chickpeas (garbanzo beans)
- ❏ cilantro
- ❏ edamame
- ❏ Fuji apple
- ❏ garlic cloves
- ❏ ginger
- ❏ grape tomatoes
- ❏ grapefruit
- ❏ green onions
- ❏ green cabbage (or Savoy cabbage)
- ❏ haricots verts
- ❏ jalapeño pepper
- ❏ leeks
- ❏ lemons
- ❏ limes
- ❏ mint
- ❏ Napa cabbage
- ❏ nectarines
- ❏ onions
- ❏ oregano
- ❏ parsley, flat-leaf
- ❏ peach
- ❏ purple sweet potato
- ❏ red bell peppers
- ❏ red onions
- ❏ red potato
- ❏ rosemary
- ❏ sage
- ❏ serrano chile
- ❏ shallots
- ❏ shiitake mushrooms
- ❏ strawberries
- ❏ sweet potatoes
- ❏ tarragon
- ❏ thyme

Baking/Cooking Products

- ❏ baking powder
- ❏ baking soda
- ❏ baking spray with flour (such as Baker's Joy®)
- ❏ brown sugar
- ❏ canola oil
- ❏ cornstarch
- ❏ dark sesame oil
- ❏ flour, all-purpose
- ❏ nonstick cooking spray
- ❏ olive oil, extra-virgin
- ❏ panko (Japanese breadcrumbs)
- ❏ sesame oil
- ❏ sugar
- ❏ vanilla extract

Spices

- ❏ black pepper
- ❏ cinnamon
- ❏ coriander
- ❏ cumin
- ❏ oregano
- ❏ red pepper
- ❏ salt

Nuts/Seeds
- [ ] almonds, dry-roasted
- [ ] pumpkin seeds
- [ ] sesame seeds
- [ ] walnuts

Condiments, Spreads and Sauces
- [ ] canola mayonnaise
- [ ] cider vinegar
- [ ] Dijon mustard
- [ ] dill pickle juice
- [ ] fish sauce
- [ ] hoisin sauce
- [ ] honey
- [ ] hot sauce
- [ ] soy sauce, lower-sodium
- [ ] yellow mustard

Breads, Cereals and Pasta
- [ ] bread, multigrain
- [ ] brown rice
- [ ] Chinese-style noodles
- [ ] English muffin
- [ ] fettuccine
- [ ] French bread baguette
- [ ] hot dog buns
- [ ] oats, old-fashioned rolled
- [ ] sourdough bread
- [ ] spaghetti, whole-wheat
- [ ] wheat flakes cereal
- [ ] wonton wrappers

Canned/Frozen Foods
- [ ] baby spinach
- [ ] cannellini beans, no-salt-added
- [ ] chicken broth, fat-free, lower-sodium
- [ ] green chiles
- [ ] mushroom caps
- [ ] pie dough

Dairy Products
- [ ] butter
- [ ] buttermilk, fat-free
- [ ] margarine, light
- [ ] milk, nonfat
- [ ] Parmigiano-Reggiano cheese
- [ ] pecorino Romano cheese
- [ ] yogurt, Greek, fat-free plain
- [ ] yogurt, strawberry, fat-free

Juices
- [ ] apple cider
- [ ] guava nectar
- [ ] lemon juice
- [ ] lime juice

Meat and Poultry
- [ ] bacon
- [ ] chicken breast halves
- [ ] chicken thighs, skinless and boneless
- [ ] eggs
- [ ] flank steak
- [ ] pancetta or cured bacon
- [ ] pork loin
- [ ] salmon fillets
- [ ] shrimp
- [ ] smoked bacon

Second Week Meals and Recipes

DAY 1

Breakfast

Strawberry Guava Smoothie

1 cup strawberries, quartered
½ cup guava nectar
1 ripe banana, frozen and sliced

1 (6-oz.) carton strawberry fat-free
yogurt
5 ice cubes (about 2 oz.)

Place all ingredients in a blender and process 2 minutes or until smooth. Serve immediately. Serves 2.

Nutritional Information: 91 calories; 0g fat; 1g protein; 22g carbohydrate; 1g dietary fiber; 0mg cholesterol; 16mg sodium.

Lunch

Chicken Nuggets with Honey Mustard and Potato Chips

Chicken nuggets:

4 (6-oz.) skinless, boneless chicken
breast halves, cut into
1″ pieces
⅓ cup fat-free buttermilk
⅓ cup dill pickle juice

¼ tsp. salt
1½ cups panko (Japanese
breadcrumbs)
2 tbsp. water
1 large egg, lightly beaten

Potato chips:

1 tbsp. extra-virgin olive oil
1 medium purple sweet potato
(about 8 oz.), cut crosswise into
⅛″-thick slices

¼ tsp. salt
1 medium baking potato (about
8 oz.), cut crosswise into
⅛″-thick slices

Honey Mustard Sauce:

¼ cup canola mayonnaise
¼ cup fat-free plain Greek yogurt
1 tbsp. honey

1 tbsp. yellow mustard
1 tsp. Dijon mustard

To prepare the chicken nuggets, combine chicken, buttermilk and pickle juice in a large zip-top plastic bag. Marinate in refrigerator 1 hour, turning occasionally. Place panko in a large skillet; cook over medium heat 3 minutes or until toasted, stirring frequently. Preheat oven to 400° F. Remove chicken from marinade; discard marinade. Sprinkle chicken evenly with ¼ teaspoon salt. Place panko in a zip-top plastic bag. Combine 2 tablespoons water and egg in a shallow dish; dip half of chicken in egg mixture. Add chicken to bag; seal and shake to coat. Remove chicken from bag; arrange chicken in a single layer on a baking sheet. Repeat procedure with remaining egg mixture, panko and chicken. Bake chicken at 400° F for 12 minutes or until done. To prepare chips, combine oil and ¼ teaspoon salt in a large bowl. Add potatoes; toss gently to coat. Place microwave plate over parchment paper. Cut paper to fit plate. Cover plate with parchment paper; arrange purple potato slices in a single layer over paper. Microwave on high for 4 minutes or until potatoes are crisp and begin to brown. Repeat procedure with baking potatoes, reusing parchment paper. To prepare sauce, combine mayonnaise, yogurt, honey and mustards in a medium bowl; stir to combine. Serve with chicken nuggets and potato chips. Serves 8.

Nutritional Information: 241 calories; 6g fat; 24g protein; 21g carbohydrate; 2g dietary fiber; 76mg cholesterol; 386mg sodium.

Dinner

Seared Salmon and Spinach

4 (6-oz.) salmon fillets	1 pint grape tomatoes, halved
¾ tsp. salt, divided	3 garlic cloves, sliced
¼ tsp. black pepper, divided	1 (9-oz.) package baby spinach
1 tbsp. canola oil, divided	2 tbsp. fresh basil

Preheat oven to 450° F. Sprinkle salmon with ½ teaspoon salt and ⅛ teaspoon pepper. Heat a large cast-iron skillet over high heat. Add 2 teaspoons oil; swirl. Add fillets, skin side down; cook for 3 minutes or until skin begins to brown, gently pressing fillets. Place pan in oven. Bake at 450° F for 6 minutes or until desired degree of doneness. Heat a nonstick skillet over medium-high heat. Add 1 teaspoon oil; swirl. Add tomatoes; sauté 1 minute. Add garlic; sauté for 30 seconds, stirring constantly. Add spinach; remove from heat. Toss until spinach wilts. Stir in ¼ teaspoon salt and ⅛ teaspoon pepper. Place about ½ cup spinach mixture on each of 4 plates; top each serving with 1 fillet and basil. Serves 4.

Nutritional Information: 346 calories; 17g fat; 38g protein; 11g carbohydrate; 4g dietary fiber; 87mg cholesterol; 545mg sodium.

DAY 2

Breakfast

Greek Yogurt with Blackberries and Cinnamon Crisps

8 wonton wrappers, cut in
half diagonally
1 tbsp. sugar
¼ tsp. ground cinnamon

1½ cups plain fat-free Greek yogurt
1 cup fresh blackberries
4 tsp. honey
nonstick cooking spray

Preheat oven to 400° F. Arrange wonton wrappers in a single layer on a baking sheet coated with nonstick cooking spray; lightly coat wrappers with cooking spray. Combine sugar and cinnamon in a small bowl. Sprinkle sugar mixture evenly over wrappers; bake at 400° F for 3 minutes or until crisp and slightly browned. Set the wrappers aside to cool slightly. Layer 6 tablespoons yogurt, ¼ cup berries and 1 teaspoon honey into each of 4 bowls. Serve each with 4 wonton crisps. Serves 4.

Nutritional Information: 142 calories; 1g fat; 10g protein; 25g carbohydrate; 2g dietary fiber; 1mg cholesterol; 124mg sodium.

Lunch

Chinese Pork Lettuce Wraps

1 small green cabbage (or Savoy
   cabbage)
2 tbsp. lower-sodium soy sauce
2 tbsp. dark sesame oil
1 tbsp. hoisin sauce
1 tsp. cornstarch
1 (8-oz.) boneless pork loin, trimmed

½ cup carrots, matchstick-cut
4 mushroom caps, thinly sliced
2 tbsp. canola oil, divided
¾ cup green onions, sliced
   and divided
3 tbsp. water
2 tsp. garlic cloves, minced

Reserve 8 cabbage leaves. Shred remaining cabbage to measure 2 cups. In medium bowl, combine soy sauce, sesame oil, hoisin sauce and cornstarch; whisk until combined. Cut pork crosswise into ¼-inch-thick slices. Stack several slices vertically; slice pork into ¼-inch-thick pieces. Repeat procedure with remaining pork. Add pork, carrots and mushrooms to soy sauce mixture; toss. Heat a large skillet over medium-high heat. Add 1 tablespoon oil. Add ¼ cup onions; sauté 30 seconds. Add shredded cabbage and water; sauté 2 minutes. Remove cabbage mixture from pan. Add remaining 1 tablespoon oil. Add remaining ½ cup onions and garlic; sauté 30 seconds. Add pork mixture; sauté 3 minutes or until done. Add cabbage mixture; toss. Place about ⅓ cup pork mixture into each of 8 reserved cabbage leaves. Serves 4.

Nutritional Information: 248 calories; 17g fat; 14g protein; 12g carbohydrate; 4g dietary fiber; 33mg cholesterol; 386mg sodium.

Dinner

Potato, Chicken and Leek Pot Pie

1 slice smoked bacon, chopped
1½ cups red potato (about 8 oz.), cubed
1 cup carrots, chopped
6 skinless, boneless chicken thighs, cut into bite-sized pieces
3½ tbsp. all-purpose flour
3 cups leeks (about 2), sliced

½ tsp. salt
¼ tsp. black pepper
2 cups fat-free, lower-sodium chicken broth
½ (14-oz.) package refrigerated pie dough
1 tbsp. nonfat milk
1 large egg white

Preheat oven to 450° F. Cook bacon in a large Dutch oven over medium heat until almost crisp, stirring frequently. Increase heat to medium-high. Add potato and carrot to pan; sauté 3 minutes, stirring occasionally. Add chicken; sauté 3 minutes or until lightly browned, stirring occasionally. Stir in flour, leeks, salt and pepper; sauté 1 minute, stirring frequently. Slowly add broth to pan, stirring constantly; bring to a boil. Cook 2 minutes or until slightly thick, stirring occasionally. Spoon mixture into a 1½-quart glass or ceramic baking dish. Top with dough, folding under and pressing down on edges to seal. Combine milk and egg white; brush mixture over top of dough. Cut small slits in dough to vent. Bake at 450° F for 30 minutes or until crust is golden. Let stand 10 minutes. Serves 6.

Nutritional Information: 298 calories; 12g fat; 18g protein; 31g carbohydrate; 2g dietary fiber; 62mg cholesterol; 561mg sodium.

DAY 3

Breakfast

1 cup wheat flakes cereal
1 cup nonfat milk

1 medium peach, sliced

Nutritional Information: 253 calories; 3g fat; 18g protein; 60g carbohydrate; 27g dietary fiber; 4mg cholesterol; 127mg sodium.

Lunch

Chicken and Rice Summer Salad

3 (6-oz.) skinless, boneless chicken
breast halves, trimmed
1 tsp. salt, divided
½ tsp. black pepper, divided
2 tbsp. extra-virgin olive oil
1 tsp. lemon rind, grated
2 tbsp. lemon juice
2 tsp. Dijon mustard
1 ½ cups nectarines, pitted and
coarsely chopped

1 cup brown rice, cooked
and cooled
1 cup cherries, pitted and coarsely
chopped
½ cup green onions, sliced
2 cups lettuce (such as arugula or
watercress), chopped
¼ cup dry-roasted almonds, chopped
3 tbsp. mint, torn
nonstick cooking spray

Preheat grill to medium-high heat. Sprinkle both sides of chicken evenly with ½ teaspoon salt and ¼ teaspoon pepper. Place chicken on a grill rack coated with nonstick cooking spray; grill 5 minutes on each side or until done. Let stand 5 minutes. Chop chicken. Combine oil, rind, juice and mustard in a large bowl, stirring well with a whisk. Add chicken, nectarines, rice, cherries, onions, lettuce, almonds and mint; toss well. Serves 4.

Nutritional Information: 299 calories; 11g fat; 23g protein; 27g carbohydrate; 4g dietary fiber; 49mg cholesterol; 705mg sodium.

Dinner

Steak Sandwich with Pickled Onions

¼ cup water
¼ cup cider vinegar
2 tbsp. sugar
1 cup red onion, thinly sliced
¼ cup canola mayonnaise
1 tbsp. fresh thyme, chopped
1 tbsp. fresh tarragon, chopped
1 tbsp. lemon juice

1 garlic clove, minced
1 lb. flank steak, trimmed
1½ tsp. extra-virgin olive oil
¼ tsp. salt
¼ tsp. black pepper
1 (12-oz.) French bread baguette
1 cup arugula

Combine water, vinegar and sugar in a medium microwave-safe bowl; microwave on high for 2 minutes or until boiling. Stir in onion. Let stand at room temperature for 30 minutes. Preheat grill to medium-high heat. In a small bowl, combine mayonnaise, thyme, tarragon, lemon juice and garlic. Rub steak evenly with oil; sprinkle with salt and pepper. Place steak on grill rack; grill 5 minutes on each side or until desired degree of doneness. Remove from grill; let stand 5 minutes. Cut steak across the grain into thin slices. Cut baguette in half lengthwise. Hollow out top and bottom halves of bread, leaving a ½-inch-thick shell; reserve torn bread for another use. Place bread, cut sides down, on grill rack; grill 1 minute or until toasted. Drain onion mixture; discard liquid. Arrange steak evenly over bottom half of baguette; top evenly with onion and arugula. Spread mayonnaise mixture over cut side of top baguette half; place on sandwich. Cut into 4 pieces. Serves 4.

Nutritional Information: 403 calories; 12g fat; 30g protein; 43g carbohydrate; 2g dietary fiber; 37mg cholesterol; 677mg sodium.

DAY 4

Breakfast

Streusel Nut Bread
Streusel:
⅓ cup brown sugar, packed
⅓ cup old-fashioned
  rolled oats
1 tbsp. all-purpose flour

¼ tsp. ground cinnamon
dash of salt
2 tbsp. butter, melted
2 tbsp. walnuts, chopped

Bread:
9 oz. all-purpose flour
  (about 2 cups)
½ tsp. baking soda
½ tsp. baking powder
½ tsp. salt
5 tbsp. butter, softened

⅔ cup sugar
3 large eggs
1 tsp. vanilla extract
1 cup fat-free buttermilk
baking spray with flour (such
  as Baker's Joy®)

Preheat oven to 350° F. To prepare streusel, combine brown sugar, oats, flour, cinnamon and salt in a medium bowl. Add 2 tablespoons melted butter, stirring until well combined. Stir in nuts. Set aside. To prepare bread, weigh or lightly spoon 9 ounces of flour into dry measuring cups; level with a knife. Combine flour, baking soda, baking powder and ½ teaspoon salt in a bowl, stirring well with a whisk. Combine 5 tablespoons butter and granulated sugar in a large bowl; beat with a mixer at medium-high speed until well blended. Add eggs, 1 at a time, beating well after each addition; beat in vanilla. Beating at low speed, add flour mixture and buttermilk alternately to sugar mixture, beginning and ending with flour mixture; beat just until combined. Scrape half of batter into a 9" x 5" loaf pan coated with baking spray; sprinkle with half of streusel mixture. Spread remaining batter over streusel; swirl. Sprinkle remaining streusel on top of batter. Bake at 350° F for 50 minutes or until a wooden pick inserted in center comes out with moist crumbs clinging. Cool 10 minutes in pan on a wire rack. Remove from pan; cool completely on wire rack. Serves 16.

Nutritional Information: 187 calories; 7g fat; 4g protein; 28g carbohydrate; 1g dietary fiber; 47mg cholesterol; 200mg sodium.

Lunch

White Chicken Chili

1 tbsp. canola oil
1 lb. skinless, boneless chicken breast, cubed
¾ tsp. salt, divided
½ cup onion, vertically sliced
2 tsp. garlic cloves, minced
2 tsp. ground cumin
1 tsp. ground coriander
½ tsp. dried oregano

¼ tsp. ground red pepper
3 cups no-salt-added canned cannellini beans, rinsed and drained
1 cup water
2 (4-oz.) cans green chiles, undrained
1 (14-oz.) can fat-free, lower-sodium chicken broth
¼ cup fresh cilantro
1 lime, cut into 8 wedges

Heat a Dutch oven over medium-high heat. Add oil. Sprinkle chicken with ¼ teaspoon salt. Add chicken; sauté 4 minutes. Add onion, garlic, cumin, coriander, oregano and red pepper; sauté 3 minutes. Add 2 cups beans, water, ½ teaspoon salt, 1 can chiles and broth; bring to a boil. Mash 1 cup beans and 1 can chiles in a bowl. Add to soup; simmer 5 minutes. Serve with cilantro and lime wedges. Serves 6.

Nutritional Information: 189 calories; 4g fat; 22g protein; 15g carbohydrate; 5g dietary fiber; 44mg cholesterol; 624mg sodium.

Dinner

Roasted Tomatoes and Garlic with Pasta

1 tbsp. plus ½ tsp. salt
¼ cup fresh basil
8 oz. whole-wheat spaghetti, uncooked
¼ cup extra-virgin olive oil, divided

2 pints multicolored cherry tomatoes
4 garlic cloves, thinly sliced
¼ tsp. black pepper
2 oz. Parmigiano-Reggiano cheese, shaved

Preheat oven to 450° F. Bring a large pot of water to a boil; add 1 tablespoon salt. Add pasta; cook 8 to 10 minutes or until *al dente*. Drain pasta in a colander over a bowl, reserving 6 tablespoons cooking liquid. Return pasta to pan. Combine reserved cooking liquid and 2 tablespoons oil in a small saucepan; bring to a boil. Boil 4 minutes or until mixture measures ⅓ cup. Add oil mixture to pan with pasta; toss to coat. While pasta cooks, combine remaining 2 tablespoons oil, tomatoes and garlic on a jelly-roll pan, tossing to combine. Bake at 450° F for 11 minutes or until tomatoes are lightly browned and begin to burst. Add tomato mixture, ½ teaspoon salt and pepper to pasta; toss to coat. Top with cheese and basil. Serves 4.

Nutritional Information: 417 calories; 18g fat; 14g protein; 50g carbohydrate; 4g dietary fiber; 10mg cholesterol; 596mg sodium.

DAY 5

Breakfast
1 (2-oz.) English muffin
1 tsp. light margarine

½ medium grapefruit
1 cup nonfat milk

Nutritional Information: 273 calories; 3g fat; 13g protein; 48g carbohydrate; 3g dietary fiber; 4mg cholesterol; 435mg sodium.

Lunch
Three Bean Salad
1 medium red bell pepper
¾ cup edamame (green soybeans), shelled
8 oz. haricots verts, trimmed
1½ cups fresh chickpeas (garbanzo beans), cooked and shelled
½ tsp. salt

½ tsp. black pepper
¼ cup shallots, minced
3 tbsp. fresh flat-leaf parsley
1½ tbsp. fresh oregano
2 tbsp. lemon juice
1 tbsp. Dijon mustard
1 tbsp. extra-virgin olive oil

Preheat broiler to high. Cut bell pepper in half lengthwise; discard seeds and membranes. Place pepper halves, skin sides up, on a foil-lined baking sheet; flatten with hand. Broil for 10 minutes or until blackened. Place in a paper bag; fold to close tightly. Let stand 10 minutes. Peel and chop. Cook edamame and haricots verts in boiling water 4 minutes; rinse with cold water and drain. Combine bell pepper, edamame mixture, chickpeas, salt and pepper in a medium bowl. In small bowl, combine shallots, parsley, oregano, lemon juice mustard and oil, stirring well with a whisk. Drizzle dressing over bean mixture; toss. Serves 6.

Nutritional Information: 255 calories; 6g fat; 13g protein; 39g carbohydrate; 12g dietary fiber; 0mg cholesterol; 245mg sodium.

Dinner

Apple and Rosemary Pork Roll

1 tsp. extra-virgin olive oil
¾ cup onion, pre-chopped
¾ cup Fuji apple, chopped
2 tsp. garlic cloves, minced
1 tbsp. cider vinegar
1 tsp. fresh rosemary, chopped
1 (1-lb.) pork loin, trimmed

½ tsp. salt, divided
¼ tsp. black pepper
⅓ cup fat-free, lower-sodium
  chicken broth
3 tbsp. apple cider
1 tsp. Dijon mustard
nonstick cooking spray

Preheat oven to 425° F. Heat a large ovenproof skillet over medium-high heat. Add oil; swirl to coat. Add onion, apple and garlic; sauté 5 minutes or until tender. Add vinegar and rosemary; cook 1 minute. Place apple mixture in a small bowl. Wipe pan clean. Slice pork lengthwise, cutting to (but not through) the other side. Open halves, laying pork flat. Starting from the center, slice each half lengthwise, cutting to (but not through) other side; open so pork is flat. Place plastic wrap over pork; pound to an even thickness using a meat mallet or small heavy skillet. Sprinkle evenly with ⅜ teaspoon salt and pepper. Spread apple mixture on pork. Roll up, jelly-roll fashion. Return pan to medium-high heat. Coat pan with nonstick cooking spray. Add pork, seam side down; cook 4 minutes or until browned, carefully turning occasionally. Place pan in oven. Bake at 425° F for 15 minutes or until a thermometer inserted in the center registers 145° F. Remove pork from pan; let stand 5 minutes before slicing. Return pan to medium-high heat; add stock, cider, mustard and remaining ⅛ teaspoon salt, stirring with a whisk. Bring to a boil; cook 2 minutes. Serve over pork. Serves 4.

Nutritional Information: 181 calories; 4g fat; 25g protein; 10g carbohydrate; 1g dietary fiber; 74mg cholesterol; 343mg sodium.

DAY 6

Breakfast

2 slices sourdough bread,
  toasted and topped with 1 tsp.
  light margarine

¾ cup blueberries
1 cup nonfat milk

Nutritional Information: 304 calories; 4g fat; 13g protein; 53g carbohydrate; 4g dietary fiber; 4mg cholesterol; 483mg sodium.

Lunch

Cabbage Salad with Grilled Sweet Potatoes

3 medium sweet potatoes (2 lbs.)
5 tbsp. extra-virgin olive oil, divided
¾ tsp. salt, divided
½ tsp. black pepper, divided
¼ cup lime juice
2 tbsp. warm water
2 tsp. honey

dash of hot sauce (optional)
1 jalapeño pepper, seeded and minced
3 cups Napa cabbage, shredded
1 cup red onion, sliced
⅓ cup pumpkin seeds, toasted
¼ cup green onions, chopped
¼ cup fresh cilantro, chopped

Prepare grill for indirect grilling, heating one side to medium-high and leaving one side with no heat. Peel potatoes and cut lengthwise into ½″ thick slices. Combine potatoes, 1 tablespoon oil, ¼ teaspoon salt and ¼ teaspoon black pepper; toss. Place potatoes on grill rack over unheated side; close lid. Cook 12 minutes on each side or until tender. Move potatoes to heated side; grill 2 minutes on each side or until charred. In a large bowl combine remaining ¼ cup oil, ½ teaspoon salt, ¼ teaspoon black pepper, juice, water, honey, hot sauce and jalapeño pepper. Cut potato slices into strips. Add potatoes, cabbage, red onion, pumpkin seeds, green onion and cilantro to large bowl; toss. Serves 6.

Nutritional Information: 259 calories; 12g fat; 4g protein; 35g carbohydrate; 6g dietary fiber; 0mg cholesterol; 330mg sodium.

Dinner

Sesame Chicken with Noodles

4 shiitake mushrooms
1 cup fat-free, lower-sodium chicken broth
1 cup water
4 tsp. lower-sodium soy sauce
2 tsp. fish sauce
2 garlic cloves, crushed
1 serrano chile, thinly sliced
1 (2″) piece fresh ginger, sliced
1 quart water

2 cups uncooked Chinese-style noodles
1 lb. chicken breast cutlets
¼ tsp. black pepper
⅓ cup sesame seeds, toasted
2 tsp. sesame oil
4 baby bok choy, cut lengthwise
½ cup (¼″-thick) slices red bell pepper
1 lime, cut into 8 wedges

Remove mushroom stems. Thinly slice caps and set aside. In medium saucepan, bring stems, broth, water, soy sauce, fish sauce, cloves, ginger and chile to a boil. Remove pan from heat. Bring 1 quart of water to a boil in a large saucepan. Add noodles; cook 3 minutes or until done. Drain and set aside. Sprinkle chicken with black pepper. Place sesame seeds in a dish. Press seeds into both sides of chicken. Heat a nonstick skillet over medium-high heat. Add oil; swirl to coat. Add chicken; cook 3 minutes on each side or until done. Remove from pan. Add bok choy, cut sides down; cook 3 minutes or until browned. Add reserved mushroom slices and bell pepper. Strain broth mixture through a sieve into pan; cover and cook 2 minutes. Remove vegetables with a slotted spoon. Thinly slice chicken. Place ½ cup noodles, about ¼ cup vegetables, and 4 ounces chicken into 4 shallow bowls. Spoon ¼ cup broth mixture over each. Garnish each with two lime wedges. Serves 4.

Nutritional Information: 338 calories; 9g fat; 34g protein; 30g carbohydrate; 4g dietary fiber; 71mg cholesterol; 795mg sodium.

DAY 7

Breakfast

Egg in a Hole

1 slice bacon
4 (1-oz.) slices multigrain bread,
　lightly toasted
4 large eggs

4 tsp. fresh pecorino Romano cheese
　(about ¼ oz.), grated
1 tsp. fresh sage, chopped
¼ tsp. black pepper

Position an oven rack in the middle setting. Place a jelly-roll pan on rack. Preheat oven to 400° F. Place bacon on heated pan and cook until crisp (about 4 minutes); crumble. Cut a hole into the center of each toast using a 3″ biscuit cutter or round cookie cutter. Reserve cutouts. Arrange bread slices on hot pan; crack one egg into each hole. Sprinkle eggs evenly with crumbled bacon, cheese and sage. Bake at 400° F for 5 minutes or until egg whites are set. Sprinkle with pepper and serve with toasted cutout. Serves 4.

Nutritional Information: 167 calories; 8g fat; 11g protein; 13g carbohydrate; 2g dietary fiber; 216mg cholesterol; 273mg sodium.

Lunch

Shrimp Salad Hoagie

1 tbsp. butter
20 large shrimp, peeled and deveined
　(about 1 lb.)
¼ cup canola mayonnaise
1 tsp. lemon rind, grated
1 tbsp. lemon juice

2 tsp. fresh flat-leaf parsley, chopped
1½ tsp. fresh tarragon, chopped
½ tsp. black pepper
¼ tsp. salt
4 (1½-oz.) hot dog buns
8 Boston lettuce leaves

Preheat broiler to high. Heat butter in a large nonstick skillet over medium-high heat; swirl to coat. Add shrimp to pan; sauté 4 minutes or until done. Place shrimp on a large plate; chill in refrigerator for 10 minutes. Coarsely chop shrimp. Combine chopped shrimp, mayonnaise, lemon rind and juice, parsley, tarragon, pepper and salt in a large bowl. Open buns without completely splitting; arrange, cut sides up, on a baking sheet. Broil 1 minute or until toasted. Place 2 lettuce leaves in each bun; top each serving with ½ cup shrimp mixture. Serves 4.

Nutritional Information: 370 calories; 18g fat; 27g protein; 23g carbohydrate; 1g dietary fiber; 185mg cholesterol; 616mg sodium.

Dinner

Roasted Cauliflower Fettuccine

1 head cauliflower, cut into florets
3 tbsp. water
¼ tsp. salt
¼ tsp. black pepper
4½ tsp. extra-virgin olive oil, divided
8 oz. fettuccine, uncooked
1½ tsp. lemon rind, grated

1½ oz. pancetta or cured bacon, finely chopped
1 tbsp. lemon juice
2 tsp. fresh thyme, chopped
1½ tsp. garlic cloves, minced
2 oz. Parmigiano-Reggiano cheese, shaved (about ½ cup)

Preheat oven to 400° F. Combine cauliflower, water, salt and pepper; drizzle with 2 teaspoons olive oil. Toss. Arrange mixture on a baking sheet; bake at 400° F for 40 minutes or until cauliflower is tender and golden, stirring twice. Cook pasta according to package directions, omitting salt and fat. Drain in a colander over a bowl, reserving ½ cup cooking liquid. Heat a large skillet over medium heat. Add pancetta to pan and cook for 5 minutes or until crisp, stirring frequently. Remove pancetta; set aside. Add remaining 2½ teaspoons oil to drippings in pan. Add ½ cup reserved cooking liquid to drippings in pan; bring to a boil over high heat. Boil 30 seconds or until emulsified, stirring constantly with a whisk. Add rind, juice, thyme and garlic to pan. Add pasta; toss. Remove from heat. Add cauliflower and pancetta; toss. Top with cheese. Serve immediately. Serves 4.

Nutritional Information: 410 calories; 14g fat; 19g protein; 56g carbohydrate; 8g dietary fiber; 20mg cholesterol; 583mg sodium.

Member Survey

Please answer the following questions to help your leader plan your First Place 4 Health meetings so that your needs might be met in this session. Give this form to your leader at the first group meeting.

Name _____ Birth date _____

Please list those who live in your household.

Name	Relationship	Age

What church do you attend? _____

Are you interested in receiving more information about our church?

      Yes   No

Occupation _____

What talent or area of expertise would you be willing to share with our class?

_____

Why did you join First Place 4 Health?

_____

With notice, would you be willing to lead a Bible study discussion one week?

      Yes   No

Are you comfortable praying out loud? _____

If the assistant leader were absent, would you be willing to assist in weighing in members and possibly evaluating the Live It Trackers?

      Yes   No

Any other comments:

_____

_____

Personal Weight and Measurement Record

Week	Weight	+ or -	Goal this Session	Pounds to goal
1				
2				
3				
4				
5				
6				
7				
8				
9				
10				
11				
12				

Beginning Measurements

Waist _____ Hips _____ Thighs _____ Chest _____

Ending Measurements

Waist _____ Hips _____ Thighs _____ Chest _____

First Place 4 Health
Prayer Partner

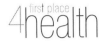

Scripture Verse to Memorize for Week Two:

Now the Lord is the Spirit, and where the Spirit of the Lord is, there is freedom.

2 Corinthians 3:17

Date: _____

Name: _____

Home Phone: (_____) _____

Work Phone: (_____) _____

Email: _____

Personal Prayer Concerns:

_____

_____

_____

_____

_____

_____

_____

This form is for prayer requests that are personal to you and your journey in First Place 4 Health. Please complete this form and have it ready to turn in when you arrive at your group meeting.

First Place 4 Health
Prayer Partner

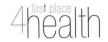

SCRIPTURE VERSE TO MEMORIZE FOR WEEK THREE:

But you are a chosen people, a royal priesthood, a holy nation,
a people belonging to God, that you may declare the praises of him who called you
out of darkness into his wonderful light.

1 PETER 2:9

Date: _____

Name: _____

Home Phone: (_____)_____

Work Phone: (_____)_____

Email: _____

Personal Prayer Concerns:

_____

_____

_____

_____

_____

_____

_____

This form is for prayer requests that are personal to you and your journey in First Place 4 Health. Please complete this form and have it ready to turn in when you arrive at your group meeting.

First Place 4 Health
Prayer Partner

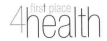

START LOSING
START LIVING
Week
3

SCRIPTURE VERSE TO MEMORIZE FOR WEEK FOUR:

And whatever you do, whether in word or deed, do it all in the name of the Lord Jesus, giving thanks to God the Father through him.

COLOSSIANS 3:17

Date: _____

Name: _____

Home Phone: (_____) _____

Work Phone: (_____) _____

Email: _____

Personal Prayer Concerns:

_____

_____

_____

_____

_____

_____

_____

This form is for prayer requests that are personal to you and your journey in First Place 4 Health. Please complete this form and have it ready to turn in when you arrive at your group meeting.

First Place 4 Health
Prayer Partner

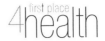

START LOSING
START LIVING
Week
4

SCRIPTURE VERSE TO MEMORIZE FOR WEEK FIVE:

But the fruit of the Spirit is love, joy, peace, patience, kindness, goodness, faithfulness, gentleness and self-control. Against such things there is no law.

GALATIANS 5:22-23

Date: _____

Name: _____

Home Phone: (_____) _____

Work Phone: (_____) _____

Email: _____

Personal Prayer Concerns:

_____

_____

_____

_____

_____

_____

_____

This form is for prayer requests that are personal to you and your journey in First Place 4 Health. Please complete this form and have it ready to turn in when you arrive at your group meeting.

First Place 4 Health
Prayer Partner

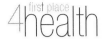

Scripture Verse to Memorize for Week Six:

Submit yourselves, then, to God. Resist the devil, and he will flee from you.

James 4:7

Date: _____

Name: _____

Home Phone: (_____) _____

Work Phone: (_____) _____

Email: _____

Personal Prayer Concerns:

_____

_____

_____

_____

_____

_____

_____

This form is for prayer requests that are personal to you and your journey in First Place 4 Health. Please complete this form and have it ready to turn in when you arrive at your group meeting.

First Place 4 Health
Prayer Partner

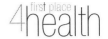

SCRIPTURE VERSE TO MEMORIZE FOR WEEK SEVEN:

*Therefore, since we are surrounded by such a great cloud of witnesses,
let us throw off everything that hinders and the sin that so easily entangles, and let
us run with perseverance the race marked out for us.*

HEBREWS 12:1

Date: _____

Name: _____

Home Phone: (_____) _____

Work Phone: (_____) _____

Email: _____

Personal Prayer Concerns:

_____

_____

_____

_____

_____

_____

_____

This form is for prayer requests that are personal to you and your journey in First Place 4 Health. Please complete this form and have it ready to turn in when you arrive at your group meeting.

First Place 4 Health
Prayer Partner

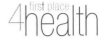

START LOSING
START LIVING
Week
7

SCRIPTURE VERSE TO MEMORIZE FOR WEEK EIGHT:

Let the word of Christ dwell in you richly as you teach and admonish
one another with all wisdom, and as you sing psalms, hymns and spiritual songs
with gratitude in your hearts to God.

COLOSSIANS 3:16

Date: _____

Name: _____

Home Phone: (_____) _____

Work Phone: (_____) _____

Email: _____

Personal Prayer Concerns:

_____

_____

_____

_____

_____

_____

_____

This form is for prayer requests that are personal to you and your journey in First Place 4 Health. Please complete this form and have it ready to turn in when you arrive at your group meeting.

First Place 4 Health
Prayer Partner

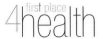

START LOSING
START LIVING
Week
8

SCRIPTURE VERSE TO MEMORIZE FOR WEEK NINE:

*Those who know your name will trust in you, for you, LORD,
have never forsaken those who seek you.*

PSALM 9:10

Date: _____

Name: _____

Home Phone: (_____) _____

Work Phone: (_____) _____

Email: _____

Personal Prayer Concerns:

_____

_____

_____

_____

_____

_____

_____

This form is for prayer requests that are personal to you and your journey in First Place 4 Health. Please complete this form and have it ready to turn in when you arrive at your group meeting.

First Place 4 Health
Prayer Partner

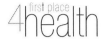

SCRIPTURE VERSE TO MEMORIZE FOR WEEK TEN:

That at the name of Jesus every knee should bow, in heaven and on earth and under the earth, and every tongue confess that Jesus Christ is Lord, to the glory of God the Father.

PHILIPPIANS 2:10-11

Date: _____

Name: _____

Home Phone: (_____) _____

Work Phone: (_____) _____

Email: _____

Personal Prayer Concerns:

_____

_____

_____

_____

_____

_____

_____

This form is for prayer requests that are personal to you and your journey in First Place 4 Health. Please complete this form and have it ready to turn in when you arrive at your group meeting.

First Place 4 Health
Prayer Partner

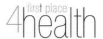

START LOSING
START LIVING
Week
10

SCRIPTURE VERSE TO MEMORIZE FOR WEEK ELEVEN:

The LORD your God is with you, he is mighty to save. He will take great delight in you,
he will quiet you with his love, he will rejoice over you with singing.

ZEPHANIAH 3:17

Date: _____

Name: _____

Home Phone: (_____) _____

Work Phone: (_____) _____

Email: _____

Personal Prayer Concerns:

_____

_____

_____

_____

_____

_____

_____

This form is for prayer requests that are personal to you and your journey in First Place 4 Health. Please complete this form and have it ready to turn in when you arrive at your group meeting.

First Place 4 Health
Prayer Partner

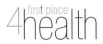

START LOSING
START LIVING
Week
11

Date: _____

Name: _____

Home Phone: (_____) _____

Work Phone: (_____) _____

Email: _____

Personal Prayer Concerns:

_____

_____

_____

_____

_____

_____

_____

This form is for prayer requests that are personal to you and your journey in First Place 4 Health. Please complete this form and have it ready to turn in when you arrive at your group meeting.

Live It Tracker

Name: _____ Date: _____ Week #: _____

Loss/gain _____ lbs.   Calorie Range: _____   My food goal for the week: _____

_____

Activity Level: None,   < 30 min/day,   30-60 min/day,   60+ min/day   My activity goal for the week: _____

My spiritual goal for the week: _____

Group	Daily Calories							
	1300-1400	1500-1600	1700-1800	1900-2000	2100-2200	2300-2400	2500-2600	2700-2800
Fruits	1.5-2 c.	1.5-2 c.	1.5-2 c.	2-2.5 c.	2-2.5 c.	2.5-3.5 c.	3.5-4.5 c.	3.5-4.5 c.
Vegetables	1.5-2 c.	2-2.5 c.	2.5-3 c.	2.5-3 c.	3-3.5 c.	3.5-4.5 c.	4.5-5 c.	4.5-5 c.
Grains	5 oz-eq.	5-6 oz-eq.	6-7 oz-eq.	6-7 oz-eq.	7-8 oz-eq.	8-9 oz-eq.	9-10 oz-eq.	10-11 oz-eq.
Meat & Beans	4 oz-eq.	5 oz-eq.	5-5.5 oz-eq.	5.5-6.5 oz-eq.	6.5-7 oz-eq.	7-7.5 oz-eq.	7-7.5 oz-eq.	7.5-8 oz-eq.
Milk	2-3 c.	3 c.	3 c.	3 c.	3 c.	3 c.	3 c.	3 c.
Healthy Oils	4 tsp.	5 tsp.	5 tsp.	6 tsp.	6 tsp.	7 tsp.	8 tsp.	8 tsp.

Day/Date:

Breakfast: _____

Lunch: _____

Dinner: _____

Snacks: _____

GROUP	FRUITS	VEGETABLES	GRAINS	MEAT & BEANS	MILK	OILS
Goal Amount						
Estimate Your Total						
Total Calories						

Physical Activity: _____   Spiritual Activity: _____

Steps/Miles/Minutes: _____   My Emotions Today: ❏ Happy   ❏ Sad   ❏ Stressed

Day/Date:

Breakfast: _____

Lunch: _____

Dinner: _____

Snacks: _____

GROUP	FRUITS	VEGETABLES	GRAINS	MEAT & BEANS	MILK	OILS
Goal Amount						
Estimate Your Total						
Total Calories						

Physical Activity: _____   Spiritual Activity: _____

Steps/Miles/Minutes: _____   My Emotions Today: ❏ Happy   ❏ Sad   ❏ Stressed

Day/Date:

Breakfast: _____

Lunch: _____

Dinner: _____

Snacks: _____

GROUP	FRUITS	VEGETABLES	GRAINS	MEAT & BEANS	MILK	OILS
Goal Amount						
Estimate Your Total						
Total Calories						

Physical Activity: _____   Spiritual Activity: _____

Steps/Miles/Minutes: _____   My Emotions Today: ❏ Happy   ❏ Sad   ❏ Stressed

Day/Date:

Breakfast: _____

Lunch: _____

Dinner: _____

Snacks: _____

GROUP	FRUITS	VEGETABLES	GRAINS	MEAT & BEANS	MILK	OILS
Goal Amount						
Estimate Your Total						
Total Calories						

Physical Activity: _____   Spiritual Activity: _____

Steps/Miles/Minutes: _____   My Emotions Today: ❑ Happy   ❑ Sad   ❑ Stressed

---

Day/Date:

Breakfast: _____

Lunch: _____

Dinner: _____

Snacks: _____

GROUP	FRUITS	VEGETABLES	GRAINS	MEAT & BEANS	MILK	OILS
Goal Amount						
Estimate Your Total						
Total Calories						

Physical Activity: _____   Spiritual Activity: _____

Steps/Miles/Minutes: _____   My Emotions Today: ❑ Happy   ❑ Sad   ❑ Stressed

---

Day/Date:

Breakfast: _____

Lunch: _____

Dinner: _____

Snacks: _____

GROUP	FRUITS	VEGETABLES	GRAINS	MEAT & BEANS	MILK	OILS
Goal Amount						
Estimate Your Total						
Total Calories						

Physical Activity: _____   Spiritual Activity: _____

Steps/Miles/Minutes: _____   My Emotions Today: ❑ Happy   ❑ Sad   ❑ Stressed

---

Day/Date:

Breakfast: _____

Lunch: _____

Dinner: _____

Snacks: _____

GROUP	FRUITS	VEGETABLES	GRAINS	MEAT & BEANS	MILK	OILS
Goal Amount						
Estimate Your Total						
Total Calories						

Physical Activity: _____   Spiritual Activity: _____

Steps/Miles/Minutes: _____   My Emotions Today: ❑ Happy   ❑ Sad   ❑ Stressed

Live It Tracker

Name: _____ Date: _____ Week #: _____

Loss/gain _____ lbs. Calorie Range: _____ My food goal for the week: _____

_____

Activity Level: None, < 30 min/day, 30-60 min/day, 60+ min/day   My activity goal for the week: _____

My spiritual goal for the week: _____

Group	Daily Calories							
	1300-1400	1500-1600	1700-1800	1900-2000	2100-2200	2300-2400	2500-2600	2700-2800
Fruits	1.5-2 c.	1.5-2 c.	1.5-2 c.	2-2.5 c.	2-2.5 c.	2.5-3.5 c.	3.5-4.5 c.	3.5-4.5 c.
Vegetables	1.5-2 c.	2-2.5 c.	2.5-3 c.	2.5-3 c.	3-3.5 c.	3.5-4.5 c.	4.5-5 c.	4.5-5 c.
Grains	5 oz-eq.	5-6 oz-eq.	6-7 oz-eq.	6-7 oz-eq.	7-8 oz-eq.	8-9 oz-eq.	9-10 oz-eq.	10-11 oz-eq.
Meat & Beans	4 oz-eq.	5 oz-eq.	5-5.5 oz-eq.	5.5-6.5 oz-eq.	6.5-7 oz-eq.	7-7.5 oz-eq.	7-7.5 oz-eq.	7.5-8 oz-eq.
Milk	2-3 c.	3 c.	3 c.	3 c.	3 c.	3 c.	3 c.	3 c.
Healthy Oils	4 tsp.	5 tsp.	5 tsp.	6 tsp.	6 tsp.	7 tsp.	8 tsp.	8 tsp.

Day/Date:

Breakfast: _____
Lunch: _____
Dinner: _____
Snacks: _____

GROUP	FRUITS	VEGETABLES	GRAINS	MEAT & BEANS	MILK	OILS
Goal Amount						
Estimate Your Total						
Total Calories						

Physical Activity: _____ Spiritual Activity: _____
Steps/Miles/Minutes: _____ My Emotions Today: ❏ Happy ❏ Sad ❏ Stressed

Day/Date:

Breakfast: _____
Lunch: _____
Dinner: _____
Snacks: _____

GROUP	FRUITS	VEGETABLES	GRAINS	MEAT & BEANS	MILK	OILS
Goal Amount						
Estimate Your Total						
Total Calories						

Physical Activity: _____ Spiritual Activity: _____
Steps/Miles/Minutes: _____ My Emotions Today: ❏ Happy ❏ Sad ❏ Stressed

Day/Date:

Breakfast: _____
Lunch: _____
Dinner: _____
Snacks: _____

GROUP	FRUITS	VEGETABLES	GRAINS	MEAT & BEANS	MILK	OILS
Goal Amount						
Estimate Your Total						
Total Calories						

Physical Activity: _____ Spiritual Activity: _____
Steps/Miles/Minutes: _____ My Emotions Today: ❏ Happy ❏ Sad ❏ Stressed

Day/Date:

Breakfast: _____

Lunch: _____

Dinner: _____

Snacks: _____

GROUP	FRUITS	VEGETABLES	GRAINS	MEAT & BEANS	MILK	OILS
Goal Amount						
Estimate Your Total						
Total Calories						

Physical Activity: _____ Spiritual Activity: _____

Steps/Miles/Minutes: _____ My Emotions Today: ❑ Happy ❑ Sad ❑ Stressed

---

Day/Date:

Breakfast: _____

Lunch: _____

Dinner: _____

Snacks: _____

GROUP	FRUITS	VEGETABLES	GRAINS	MEAT & BEANS	MILK	OILS
Goal Amount						
Estimate Your Total						
Total Calories						

Physical Activity: _____ Spiritual Activity: _____

Steps/Miles/Minutes: _____ My Emotions Today: ❑ Happy ❑ Sad ❑ Stressed

---

Day/Date:

Breakfast: _____

Lunch: _____

Dinner: _____

Snacks: _____

GROUP	FRUITS	VEGETABLES	GRAINS	MEAT & BEANS	MILK	OILS
Goal Amount						
Estimate Your Total						
Total Calories						

Physical Activity: _____ Spiritual Activity: _____

Steps/Miles/Minutes: _____ My Emotions Today: ❑ Happy ❑ Sad ❑ Stressed

---

Day/Date:

Breakfast: _____

Lunch: _____

Dinner: _____

Snacks: _____

GROUP	FRUITS	VEGETABLES	GRAINS	MEAT & BEANS	MILK	OILS
Goal Amount						
Estimate Your Total						
Total Calories						

Physical Activity: _____ Spiritual Activity: _____

Steps/Miles/Minutes: _____ My Emotions Today: ❑ Happy ❑ Sad ❑ Stressed

Live It Tracker

Name: _____ Date: _____ Week #: _____

Loss/gain _____ lbs.   Calorie Range: _____ My food goal for the week: _____

_____

Activity Level: None, < 30 min/day, 30-60 min/day, 60+ min/day   My activity goal for the week: _____

My spiritual goal for the week: _____

Group	Daily Calories							
	1300-1400	1500-1600	1700-1800	1900-2000	2100-2200	2300-2400	2500-2600	2700-2800
Fruits	1.5-2 c.	1.5-2 c.	1.5-2 c.	2-2.5 c.	2-2.5 c.	2.5-3.5 c.	3.5-4.5 c.	3.5-4.5 c.
Vegetables	1.5-2 c.	2-2.5 c.	2.5-3 c.	2.5-3 c.	3-3.5 c.	3.5-4.5 c.	4.5-5 c.	4.5-5 c.
Grains	5 oz-eq.	5-6 oz-eq.	6-7 oz-eq.	6-7 oz-eq.	7-8 oz-eq.	8-9 oz-eq.	9-10 oz-eq.	10-11 oz-eq.
Meat & Beans	4 oz-eq.	5 oz-eq.	5-5.5 oz-eq.	5.5-6.5 oz-eq.	6.5-7 oz-eq.	7-7.5 oz-eq.	7-7.5 oz-eq.	7.5-8 oz-eq.
Milk	2-3 c.	3 c.	3 c.	3 c.	3 c.	3 c.	3 c.	3 c.
Healthy Oils	4 tsp.	5 tsp.	5 tsp.	6 tsp.	6 tsp.	7 tsp.	8 tsp.	8 tsp.

Day/Date:

Breakfast: _____
Lunch: _____
Dinner: _____
Snacks: _____

GROUP	FRUITS	VEGETABLES	GRAINS	MEAT & BEANS	MILK	OILS
Goal Amount						
Estimate Your Total						
Total Calories						

Physical Activity: _____   Spiritual Activity: _____
Steps/Miles/Minutes: _____   My Emotions Today: ❏ Happy ❏ Sad ❏ Stressed

Day/Date:

Breakfast: _____
Lunch: _____
Dinner: _____
Snacks: _____

GROUP	FRUITS	VEGETABLES	GRAINS	MEAT & BEANS	MILK	OILS
Goal Amount						
Estimate Your Total						
Total Calories						

Physical Activity: _____   Spiritual Activity: _____
Steps/Miles/Minutes: _____   My Emotions Today: ❏ Happy ❏ Sad ❏ Stressed

Day/Date:

Breakfast: _____
Lunch: _____
Dinner: _____
Snacks: _____

GROUP	FRUITS	VEGETABLES	GRAINS	MEAT & BEANS	MILK	OILS
Goal Amount						
Estimate Your Total						
Total Calories						

Physical Activity: _____   Spiritual Activity: _____
Steps/Miles/Minutes: _____   My Emotions Today: ❏ Happy ❏ Sad ❏ Stressed

Day/Date:

Breakfast: _____
Lunch: _____
Dinner: _____
Snacks: _____

GROUP	FRUITS	VEGETABLES	GRAINS	MEAT & BEANS	MILK	OILS
Goal Amount						
Estimate Your Total						
Total Calories						

Physical Activity: _____   Spiritual Activity: _____
Steps/Miles/Minutes: _____   My Emotions Today: ❏ Happy ❏ Sad ❏ Stressed

---

Day/Date:

Breakfast: _____
Lunch: _____
Dinner: _____
Snacks: _____

GROUP	FRUITS	VEGETABLES	GRAINS	MEAT & BEANS	MILK	OILS
Goal Amount						
Estimate Your Total						
Total Calories						

Physical Activity: _____   Spiritual Activity: _____
Steps/Miles/Minutes: _____   My Emotions Today: ❏ Happy ❏ Sad ❏ Stressed

---

Day/Date:

Breakfast: _____
Lunch: _____
Dinner: _____
Snacks: _____

GROUP	FRUITS	VEGETABLES	GRAINS	MEAT & BEANS	MILK	OILS
Goal Amount						
Estimate Your Total						
Total Calories						

Physical Activity: _____   Spiritual Activity: _____
Steps/Miles/Minutes: _____   My Emotions Today: ❏ Happy ❏ Sad ❏ Stressed

---

Day/Date:

Breakfast: _____
Lunch: _____
Dinner: _____
Snacks: _____

GROUP	FRUITS	VEGETABLES	GRAINS	MEAT & BEANS	MILK	OILS
Goal Amount						
Estimate Your Total						
Total Calories						

Physical Activity: _____   Spiritual Activity: _____
Steps/Miles/Minutes: _____   My Emotions Today: ❏ Happy ❏ Sad ❏ Stressed

Live It Tracker

Name: _____ Date: _____ Week #: _____

Loss/gain _____ lbs.   Calorie Range: _____   My food goal for the week: _____

_____

Activity Level: None, < 30 min/day, 30-60 min/day, 60+ min/day   My activity goal for the week: _____

My spiritual goal for the week: _____

Group	Daily Calories							
	1300-1400	1500-1600	1700-1800	1900-2000	2100-2200	2300-2400	2500-2600	2700-2800
Fruits	1.5-2 c.	1.5-2 c.	1.5-2 c.	2-2.5 c.	2-2.5 c.	2.5-3.5 c.	3.5-4.5 c.	3.5-4.5 c.
Vegetables	1.5-2 c.	2-2.5 c.	2.5-3 c.	2.5-3 c.	3-3.5 c.	3.5-4.5 c.	4.5-5 c.	4.5-5 c.
Grains	5 oz-eq.	5-6 oz-eq.	6-7 oz-eq.	6-7 oz-eq.	7-8 oz-eq.	8-9 oz-eq.	9-10 oz-eq.	10-11 oz-eq.
Meat & Beans	4 oz-eq.	5 oz-eq.	5-5.5 oz-eq.	5.5-6.5 oz-eq.	6.5-7 oz-eq.	7-7.5 oz-eq.	7-7.5 oz-eq.	7.5-8 oz-eq.
Milk	2-3 c.	3 c.	3 c.	3 c.	3 c.	3 c.	3 c.	3 c.
Healthy Oils	4 tsp.	5 tsp.	5 tsp.	6 tsp.	6 tsp.	7 tsp.	8 tsp.	8 tsp.

Day/Date:

Breakfast: _____
Lunch: _____
Dinner: _____
Snacks: _____

GROUP	FRUITS	VEGETABLES	GRAINS	MEAT & BEANS	MILK	OILS
Goal Amount						
Estimate Your Total						
Total Calories						

Physical Activity: _____   Spiritual Activity: _____
Steps/Miles/Minutes: _____   My Emotions Today: ❑ Happy   ❑ Sad   ❑ Stressed

Day/Date:

Breakfast: _____
Lunch: _____
Dinner: _____
Snacks: _____

GROUP	FRUITS	VEGETABLES	GRAINS	MEAT & BEANS	MILK	OILS
Goal Amount						
Estimate Your Total						
Total Calories						

Physical Activity: _____   Spiritual Activity: _____
Steps/Miles/Minutes: _____   My Emotions Today: ❑ Happy   ❑ Sad   ❑ Stressed

Day/Date:

Breakfast: _____
Lunch: _____
Dinner: _____
Snacks: _____

GROUP	FRUITS	VEGETABLES	GRAINS	MEAT & BEANS	MILK	OILS
Goal Amount						
Estimate Your Total						
Total Calories						

Physical Activity: _____   Spiritual Activity: _____
Steps/Miles/Minutes: _____   My Emotions Today: ❑ Happy   ❑ Sad   ❑ Stressed

Day/Date:

Breakfast: _____
Lunch: _____
Dinner: _____
Snacks: _____

GROUP	FRUITS	VEGETABLES	GRAINS	MEAT & BEANS	MILK	OILS
Goal Amount						
Estimate Your Total						
Total Calories						

Physical Activity: _____   Spiritual Activity: _____
Steps/Miles/Minutes: _____   My Emotions Today: ❏ Happy   ❏ Sad   ❏ Stressed

---

Day/Date:

Breakfast: _____
Lunch: _____
Dinner: _____
Snacks: _____

GROUP	FRUITS	VEGETABLES	GRAINS	MEAT & BEANS	MILK	OILS
Goal Amount						
Estimate Your Total						
Total Calories						

Physical Activity: _____   Spiritual Activity: _____
Steps/Miles/Minutes: _____   My Emotions Today: ❏ Happy   ❏ Sad   ❏ Stressed

---

Day/Date:

Breakfast: _____
Lunch: _____
Dinner: _____
Snacks: _____

GROUP	FRUITS	VEGETABLES	GRAINS	MEAT & BEANS	MILK	OILS
Goal Amount						
Estimate Your Total						
Total Calories						

Physical Activity: _____   Spiritual Activity: _____
Steps/Miles/Minutes: _____   My Emotions Today: ❏ Happy   ❏ Sad   ❏ Stressed

---

Day/Date:

Breakfast: _____
Lunch: _____
Dinner: _____
Snacks: _____

GROUP	FRUITS	VEGETABLES	GRAINS	MEAT & BEANS	MILK	OILS
Goal Amount						
Estimate Your Total						
Total Calories						

Physical Activity: _____   Spiritual Activity: _____
Steps/Miles/Minutes: _____   My Emotions Today: ❏ Happy   ❏ Sad   ❏ Stressed

Live It Tracker

Name: _____ Date: _____ Week #: _____

Loss/gain _____ lbs.   Calorie Range: _____   My food goal for the week: _____
_____

Activity Level: None, < 30 min/day, 30-60 min/day, 60+ min/day   My activity goal for the week: _____
My spiritual goal for the week: _____

Group	Daily Calories							
	1300-1400	1500-1600	1700-1800	1900-2000	2100-2200	2300-2400	2500-2600	2700-2800
Fruits	1.5-2 c.	1.5-2 c.	1.5-2 c.	2-2.5 c.	2-2.5 c.	2.5-3.5 c.	3.5-4.5 c.	3.5-4.5 c.
Vegetables	1.5-2 c.	2-2.5 c.	2.5-3 c.	2.5-3 c.	3-3.5 c.	3.5-4.5 c.	4.5-5 c.	4.5-5 c.
Grains	5 oz-eq.	5-6 oz-eq.	6-7 oz-eq.	6-7 oz-eq.	7-8 oz-eq.	8-9 oz-eq.	9-10 oz-eq.	10-11 oz-eq.
Meat & Beans	4 oz-eq.	5 oz-eq.	5-5.5 oz-eq.	5.5-6.5 oz-eq.	6.5-7 oz-eq.	7-7.5 oz-eq.	7-7.5 oz-eq.	7.5-8 oz-eq.
Milk	2-3 c.	3 c.	3 c.	3 c.	3 c.	3 c.	3 c.	3 c.
Healthy Oils	4 tsp.	5 tsp.	5 tsp.	6 tsp.	6 tsp.	7 tsp.	8 tsp.	8 tsp.

Day/Date:

Breakfast: _____
Lunch: _____
Dinner: _____
Snacks: _____

GROUP	FRUITS	VEGETABLES	GRAINS	MEAT & BEANS	MILK	OILS
Goal Amount						
Estimate Your Total						
Total Calories						

Physical Activity: _____ Spiritual Activity: _____
Steps/Miles/Minutes: _____ My Emotions Today: ❑ Happy   ❑ Sad   ❑ Stressed

Day/Date:

Breakfast: _____
Lunch: _____
Dinner: _____
Snacks: _____

GROUP	FRUITS	VEGETABLES	GRAINS	MEAT & BEANS	MILK	OILS
Goal Amount						
Estimate Your Total						
Total Calories						

Physical Activity: _____ Spiritual Activity: _____
Steps/Miles/Minutes: _____ My Emotions Today: ❑ Happy   ❑ Sad   ❑ Stressed

Day/Date:

Breakfast: _____
Lunch: _____
Dinner: _____
Snacks: _____

GROUP	FRUITS	VEGETABLES	GRAINS	MEAT & BEANS	MILK	OILS
Goal Amount						
Estimate Your Total						
Total Calories						

Physical Activity: _____ Spiritual Activity: _____
Steps/Miles/Minutes: _____ My Emotions Today: ❑ Happy   ❑ Sad   ❑ Stressed

Day/Date:

Breakfast: _____

Lunch: _____

Dinner: _____

Snacks: _____

GROUP	FRUITS	VEGETABLES	GRAINS	MEAT & BEANS	MILK	OILS
Goal Amount						
Estimate Your Total						
Total Calories						

Physical Activity: _____ Spiritual Activity: _____

Steps/Miles/Minutes: _____ My Emotions Today: ❏ Happy ❏ Sad ❏ Stressed

---

Day/Date:

Breakfast: _____

Lunch: _____

Dinner: _____

Snacks: _____

GROUP	FRUITS	VEGETABLES	GRAINS	MEAT & BEANS	MILK	OILS
Goal Amount						
Estimate Your Total						
Total Calories						

Physical Activity: _____ Spiritual Activity: _____

Steps/Miles/Minutes: _____ My Emotions Today: ❏ Happy ❏ Sad ❏ Stressed

---

Day/Date:

Breakfast: _____

Lunch: _____

Dinner: _____

Snacks: _____

GROUP	FRUITS	VEGETABLES	GRAINS	MEAT & BEANS	MILK	OILS
Goal Amount						
Estimate Your Total						
Total Calories						

Physical Activity: _____ Spiritual Activity: _____

Steps/Miles/Minutes: _____ My Emotions Today: ❏ Happy ❏ Sad ❏ Stressed

---

Day/Date:

Breakfast: _____

Lunch: _____

Dinner: _____

Snacks: _____

GROUP	FRUITS	VEGETABLES	GRAINS	MEAT & BEANS	MILK	OILS
Goal Amount						
Estimate Your Total						
Total Calories						

Physical Activity: _____ Spiritual Activity: _____

Steps/Miles/Minutes: _____ My Emotions Today: ❏ Happy ❏ Sad ❏ Stressed

Live It Tracker

Name: _____ Date: _____ Week #: _____

Loss/gain _____ lbs.   Calorie Range: _____   My food goal for the week: _____

Activity Level: None, < 30 min/day, 30-60 min/day, 60+ min/day   My activity goal for the week: _____

My spiritual goal for the week: _____

Group	Daily Calories							
	1300-1400	1500-1600	1700-1800	1900-2000	2100-2200	2300-2400	2500-2600	2700-2800
Fruits	1.5-2 c.	1.5-2 c.	1.5-2 c.	2-2.5 c.	2-2.5 c.	2.5-3.5 c.	3.5-4.5 c.	3.5-4.5 c.
Vegetables	1.5-2 c.	2-2.5 c.	2.5-3 c.	2.5-3 c.	3-3.5 c.	3.5-4.5 c.	4.5-5 c.	4.5-5 c.
Grains	5 oz-eq.	5-6 oz-eq.	6-7 oz-eq.	6-7 oz-eq.	7-8 oz-eq.	8-9 oz-eq.	9-10 oz-eq.	10-11 oz-eq.
Meat & Beans	4 oz-eq.	5 oz-eq.	5-5.5 oz-eq.	5.5-6.5 oz-eq.	6.5-7 oz-eq.	7-7.5 oz-eq.	7-7.5 oz-eq.	7.5-8 oz-eq.
Milk	2-3 c.	3 c.	3 c.	3 c.	3 c.	3 c.	3 c.	3 c.
Healthy Oils	4 tsp.	5 tsp.	5 tsp.	6 tsp.	6 tsp.	7 tsp.	8 tsp.	8 tsp.

Day/Date:

Breakfast: _____
Lunch: _____
Dinner: _____
Snacks: _____

GROUP	FRUITS	VEGETABLES	GRAINS	MEAT & BEANS	MILK	OILS
Goal Amount						
Estimate Your Total						
Total Calories						

Physical Activity: _____   Spiritual Activity: _____
Steps/Miles/Minutes: _____   My Emotions Today: ❑ Happy   ❑ Sad ❑ Stressed

Day/Date:

Breakfast: _____
Lunch: _____
Dinner: _____
Snacks: _____

GROUP	FRUITS	VEGETABLES	GRAINS	MEAT & BEANS	MILK	OILS
Goal Amount						
Estimate Your Total						
Total Calories						

Physical Activity: _____   Spiritual Activity: _____
Steps/Miles/Minutes: _____   My Emotions Today: ❑ Happy   ❑ Sad ❑ Stressed

Day/Date:

Breakfast: _____
Lunch: _____
Dinner: _____
Snacks: _____

GROUP	FRUITS	VEGETABLES	GRAINS	MEAT & BEANS	MILK	OILS
Goal Amount						
Estimate Your Total						
Total Calories						

Physical Activity: _____   Spiritual Activity: _____
Steps/Miles/Minutes: _____   My Emotions Today: ❑ Happy   ❑ Sad ❑ Stressed

Day/Date:

Breakfast: _____
Lunch: _____
Dinner: _____
Snacks: _____

GROUP	FRUITS	VEGETABLES	GRAINS	MEAT & BEANS	MILK	OILS
Goal Amount						
Estimate Your Total						
Total Calories						

Physical Activity: _____   Spiritual Activity: _____
Steps/Miles/Minutes: _____   My Emotions Today: ❑ Happy ❑ Sad ❑ Stressed

Day/Date:

Breakfast: _____
Lunch: _____
Dinner: _____
Snacks: _____

GROUP	FRUITS	VEGETABLES	GRAINS	MEAT & BEANS	MILK	OILS
Goal Amount						
Estimate Your Total						
Total Calories						

Physical Activity: _____   Spiritual Activity: _____
Steps/Miles/Minutes: _____   My Emotions Today: ❑ Happy ❑ Sad ❑ Stressed

Day/Date:

Breakfast: _____
Lunch: _____
Dinner: _____
Snacks: _____

GROUP	FRUITS	VEGETABLES	GRAINS	MEAT & BEANS	MILK	OILS
Goal Amount						
Estimate Your Total						
Total Calories						

Physical Activity: _____   Spiritual Activity: _____
Steps/Miles/Minutes: _____   My Emotions Today: ❑ Happy ❑ Sad ❑ Stressed

Day/Date:

Breakfast: _____
Lunch: _____
Dinner: _____
Snacks: _____

GROUP	FRUITS	VEGETABLES	GRAINS	MEAT & BEANS	MILK	OILS
Goal Amount						
Estimate Your Total						
Total Calories						

Physical Activity: _____   Spiritual Activity: _____
Steps/Miles/Minutes: _____   My Emotions Today: ❑ Happy ❑ Sad ❑ Stressed

Live It Tracker

Name: _____ Date: _____ Week #: _____

Loss/gain _____ lbs. Calorie Range: _____ My food goal for the week: _____

Activity Level: None, < 30 min/day, 30-60 min/day, 60+ min/day My activity goal for the week: _____

My spiritual goal for the week: _____

Group	Daily Calories							
	1300-1400	1500-1600	1700-1800	1900-2000	2100-2200	2300-2400	2500-2600	2700-2800
Fruits	1.5-2 c.	1.5-2 c.	1.5-2 c.	2-2.5 c.	2-2.5 c.	2.5-3.5 c.	3.5-4.5 c.	3.5-4.5 c.
Vegetables	1.5-2 c.	2-2.5 c.	2.5-3 c.	2.5-3 c.	3-3.5 c.	3.5-4.5 c.	4.5-5 c.	4.5-5 c.
Grains	5 oz-eq.	5-6 oz-eq.	6-7 oz-eq.	6-7 oz-eq.	7-8 oz-eq.	8-9 oz-eq.	9-10 oz-eq.	10-11 oz-eq.
Meat & Beans	4 oz-eq.	5 oz-eq.	5-5.5 oz-eq.	5.5-6.5 oz-eq.	6.5-7 oz-eq.	7-7.5 oz-eq.	7-7.5 oz-eq.	7.5-8 oz-eq.
Milk	2-3 c.	3 c.	3 c.	3 c.	3 c.	3 c.	3 c.	3 c.
Healthy Oils	4 tsp.	5 tsp.	5 tsp.	6 tsp.	6 tsp.	7 tsp.	8 tsp.	8 tsp.

Day/Date:

Breakfast: _____
Lunch: _____
Dinner: _____
Snacks: _____

GROUP	FRUITS	VEGETABLES	GRAINS	MEAT & BEANS	MILK	OILS
Goal Amount						
Estimate Your Total						
Total Calories						

Physical Activity: _____ Spiritual Activity: _____
Steps/Miles/Minutes: _____ My Emotions Today: ❏ Happy ❏ Sad ❏ Stressed

Day/Date:

Breakfast: _____
Lunch: _____
Dinner: _____
Snacks: _____

GROUP	FRUITS	VEGETABLES	GRAINS	MEAT & BEANS	MILK	OILS
Goal Amount						
Estimate Your Total						
Total Calories						

Physical Activity: _____ Spiritual Activity: _____
Steps/Miles/Minutes: _____ My Emotions Today: ❏ Happy ❏ Sad ❏ Stressed

Day/Date:

Breakfast: _____
Lunch: _____
Dinner: _____
Snacks: _____

GROUP	FRUITS	VEGETABLES	GRAINS	MEAT & BEANS	MILK	OILS
Goal Amount						
Estimate Your Total						
Total Calories						

Physical Activity: _____ Spiritual Activity: _____
Steps/Miles/Minutes: _____ My Emotions Today: ❏ Happy ❏ Sad ❏ Stressed

Day/Date:

Breakfast: _____

Lunch: _____

Dinner: _____

Snacks: _____

GROUP	FRUITS	VEGETABLES	GRAINS	MEAT & BEANS	MILK	OILS
Goal Amount						
Estimate Your Total						
Total Calories						

Physical Activity: _____ Spiritual Activity: _____

Steps/Miles/Minutes: _____ My Emotions Today: ❑ Happy ❑ Sad ❑ Stressed

Day/Date:

Breakfast: _____

Lunch: _____

Dinner: _____

Snacks: _____

GROUP	FRUITS	VEGETABLES	GRAINS	MEAT & BEANS	MILK	OILS
Goal Amount						
Estimate Your Total						
Total Calories						

Physical Activity: _____ Spiritual Activity: _____

Steps/Miles/Minutes: _____ My Emotions Today: ❑ Happy ❑ Sad ❑ Stressed

Day/Date:

Breakfast: _____

Lunch: _____

Dinner: _____

Snacks: _____

GROUP	FRUITS	VEGETABLES	GRAINS	MEAT & BEANS	MILK	OILS
Goal Amount						
Estimate Your Total						
Total Calories						

Physical Activity: _____ Spiritual Activity: _____

Steps/Miles/Minutes: _____ My Emotions Today: ❑ Happy ❑ Sad ❑ Stressed

Day/Date:

Breakfast: _____

Lunch: _____

Dinner: _____

Snacks: _____

GROUP	FRUITS	VEGETABLES	GRAINS	MEAT & BEANS	MILK	OILS
Goal Amount						
Estimate Your Total						
Total Calories						

Physical Activity: _____ Spiritual Activity: _____

Steps/Miles/Minutes: _____ My Emotions Today: ❑ Happy ❑ Sad ❑ Stressed

Live It Tracker

Name: _____ Date: _____ Week #: _____

Loss/gain _____ lbs.　Calorie Range: _____　My food goal for the week: _____

_____

Activity Level: None, < 30 min/day, 30-60 min/day, 60+ min/day　My activity goal for the week: _____

My spiritual goal for the week: _____

Group	Daily Calories							
	1300-1400	1500-1600	1700-1800	1900-2000	2100-2200	2300-2400	2500-2600	2700-2800
Fruits	1.5-2 c.	1.5-2 c.	1.5-2 c.	2-2.5 c.	2-2.5 c.	2.5-3.5 c.	3.5-4.5 c.	3.5-4.5 c.
Vegetables	1.5-2 c.	2-2.5 c.	2.5-3 c.	2.5-3 c.	3-3.5 c.	3.5-4.5 c.	4.5-5 c.	4.5-5 c.
Grains	5 oz-eq.	5-6 oz-eq.	6-7 oz-eq.	6-7 oz-eq.	7-8 oz-eq.	8-9 oz-eq.	9-10 oz-eq.	10-11 oz-eq.
Meat & Beans	4 oz-eq.	5 oz-eq.	5-5.5 oz-eq.	5.5-6.5 oz-eq.	6.5-7 oz-eq.	7-7.5 oz-eq.	7-7.5 oz-eq.	7.5-8 oz-eq.
Milk	2-3 c.	3 c.	3 c.	3 c.	3 c.	3 c.	3 c.	3 c.
Healthy Oils	4 tsp.	5 tsp.	5 tsp.	6 tsp.	6 tsp.	7 tsp.	8 tsp.	8 tsp.

Day/Date:

Breakfast: _____
Lunch: _____
Dinner: _____
Snacks: _____

GROUP	FRUITS	VEGETABLES	GRAINS	MEAT & BEANS	MILK	OILS
Goal Amount						
Estimate Your Total						
Total Calories						

Physical Activity: _____　Spiritual Activity: _____
Steps/Miles/Minutes: _____　My Emotions Today: ❑ Happy　❑ Sad　❑ Stressed

Day/Date:

Breakfast: _____
Lunch: _____
Dinner: _____
Snacks: _____

GROUP	FRUITS	VEGETABLES	GRAINS	MEAT & BEANS	MILK	OILS
Goal Amount						
Estimate Your Total						
Total Calories						

Physical Activity: _____　Spiritual Activity: _____
Steps/Miles/Minutes: _____　My Emotions Today: ❑ Happy　❑ Sad　❑ Stressed

Day/Date:

Breakfast: _____
Lunch: _____
Dinner: _____
Snacks: _____

GROUP	FRUITS	VEGETABLES	GRAINS	MEAT & BEANS	MILK	OILS
Goal Amount						
Estimate Your Total						
Total Calories						

Physical Activity: _____　Spiritual Activity: _____
Steps/Miles/Minutes: _____　My Emotions Today: ❑ Happy　❑ Sad　❑ Stressed

Day/Date:

Breakfast: _____
Lunch: _____
Dinner: _____
Snacks: _____

GROUP	FRUITS	VEGETABLES	GRAINS	MEAT & BEANS	MILK	OILS
Goal Amount						
Estimate Your Total						
Total Calories						

Physical Activity: _____
Steps/Miles/Minutes: _____

Spiritual Activity: _____
My Emotions Today: ❑ Happy ❑ Sad ❑ Stressed

Day/Date:

Breakfast: _____
Lunch: _____
Dinner: _____
Snacks: _____

GROUP	FRUITS	VEGETABLES	GRAINS	MEAT & BEANS	MILK	OILS
Goal Amount						
Estimate Your Total						
Total Calories						

Physical Activity: _____
Steps/Miles/Minutes: _____

Spiritual Activity: _____
My Emotions Today: ❑ Happy ❑ Sad ❑ Stressed

Day/Date:

Breakfast: _____
Lunch: _____
Dinner: _____
Snacks: _____

GROUP	FRUITS	VEGETABLES	GRAINS	MEAT & BEANS	MILK	OILS
Goal Amount						
Estimate Your Total						
Total Calories						

Physical Activity: _____
Steps/Miles/Minutes: _____

Spiritual Activity: _____
My Emotions Today: ❑ Happy ❑ Sad ❑ Stressed

Day/Date:

Breakfast: _____
Lunch: _____
Dinner: _____
Snacks: _____

GROUP	FRUITS	VEGETABLES	GRAINS	MEAT & BEANS	MILK	OILS
Goal Amount						
Estimate Your Total						
Total Calories						

Physical Activity: _____
Steps/Miles/Minutes: _____

Spiritual Activity: _____
My Emotions Today: ❑ Happy ❑ Sad ❑ Stressed

Live It Tracker

Name: _____ Date: _____ Week #: _____

Loss/gain _____ lbs.   Calorie Range: _____   My food goal for the week: _____

_____

Activity Level: None, < 30 min/day, 30-60 min/day, 60+ min/day   My activity goal for the week: _____

My spiritual goal for the week: _____

Group	Daily Calories							
	1300-1400	1500-1600	1700-1800	1900-2000	2100-2200	2300-2400	2500-2600	2700-2800
Fruits	1.5-2 c.	1.5-2 c.	1.5-2 c.	2-2.5 c.	2-2.5 c.	2.5-3.5 c.	3.5-4.5 c.	3.5-4.5 c.
Vegetables	1.5-2 c.	2-2.5 c.	2.5-3 c.	2.5-3 c.	3-3.5 c.	3.5-4.5 c.	4.5-5 c.	4.5-5 c.
Grains	5 oz-eq.	5-6 oz-eq.	6-7 oz-eq.	6-7 oz-eq.	7-8 oz-eq.	8-9 oz-eq.	9-10 oz-eq.	10-11 oz-eq.
Meat & Beans	4 oz-eq.	5 oz-eq.	5-5.5 oz-eq.	5.5-6.5 oz-eq.	6.5-7 oz-eq.	7-7.5 oz-eq.	7-7.5 oz-eq.	7.5-8 oz-eq.
Milk	2-3 c.	3 c.	3 c.	3 c.	3 c.	3 c.	3 c.	3 c.
Healthy Oils	4 tsp.	5 tsp.	5 tsp.	6 tsp.	6 tsp.	7 tsp.	8 tsp.	8 tsp.

Day/Date:

Breakfast: _____

Lunch: _____

Dinner: _____

Snacks: _____

GROUP	FRUITS	VEGETABLES	GRAINS	MEAT & BEANS	MILK	OILS
Goal Amount						
Estimate Your Total						
Total Calories						

Physical Activity: _____   Spiritual Activity: _____

Steps/Miles/Minutes: _____   My Emotions Today: ❑ Happy ❑ Sad ❑ Stressed

Day/Date:

Breakfast: _____

Lunch: _____

Dinner: _____

Snacks: _____

GROUP	FRUITS	VEGETABLES	GRAINS	MEAT & BEANS	MILK	OILS
Goal Amount						
Estimate Your Total						
Total Calories						

Physical Activity: _____   Spiritual Activity: _____

Steps/Miles/Minutes: _____   My Emotions Today: ❑ Happy ❑ Sad ❑ Stressed

Day/Date:

Breakfast: _____

Lunch: _____

Dinner: _____

Snacks: _____

GROUP	FRUITS	VEGETABLES	GRAINS	MEAT & BEANS	MILK	OILS
Goal Amount						
Estimate Your Total						
Total Calories						

Physical Activity: _____   Spiritual Activity: _____

Steps/Miles/Minutes: _____   My Emotions Today: ❑ Happy ❑ Sad ❑ Stressed

Day/Date: _____

Breakfast: _____

Lunch: _____

Dinner: _____

Snacks: _____

GROUP	FRUITS	VEGETABLES	GRAINS	MEAT & BEANS	MILK	OILS
Goal Amount						
Estimate Your Total						
Total Calories						

Physical Activity: _____ Spiritual Activity: _____

Steps/Miles/Minutes: _____ My Emotions Today: ❏ Happy ❏ Sad ❏ Stressed

---

Day/Date: _____

Breakfast: _____

Lunch: _____

Dinner: _____

Snacks: _____

GROUP	FRUITS	VEGETABLES	GRAINS	MEAT & BEANS	MILK	OILS
Goal Amount						
Estimate Your Total						
Total Calories						

Physical Activity: _____ Spiritual Activity: _____

Steps/Miles/Minutes: _____ My Emotions Today: ❏ Happy ❏ Sad ❏ Stressed

---

Day/Date: _____

Breakfast: _____

Lunch: _____

Dinner: _____

Snacks: _____

GROUP	FRUITS	VEGETABLES	GRAINS	MEAT & BEANS	MILK	OILS
Goal Amount						
Estimate Your Total						
Total Calories						

Physical Activity: _____ Spiritual Activity: _____

Steps/Miles/Minutes: _____ My Emotions Today: ❏ Happy ❏ Sad ❏ Stressed

---

Day/Date: _____

Breakfast: _____

Lunch: _____

Dinner: _____

Snacks: _____

GROUP	FRUITS	VEGETABLES	GRAINS	MEAT & BEANS	MILK	OILS
Goal Amount						
Estimate Your Total						
Total Calories						

Physical Activity: _____ Spiritual Activity: _____

Steps/Miles/Minutes: _____ My Emotions Today: ❏ Happy ❏ Sad ❏ Stressed

Live It Tracker

Name: _____ Date: _____ Week #: _____

Loss/gain _____ lbs. Calorie Range: _____ My food goal for the week: _____

_____

Activity Level: None, < 30 min/day, 30-60 min/day, 60+ min/day   My activity goal for the week: _____

My spiritual goal for the week: _____

Group	Daily Calories							
	1300-1400	1500-1600	1700-1800	1900-2000	2100-2200	2300-2400	2500-2600	2700-2800
Fruits	1.5-2 c.	1.5-2 c.	1.5-2 c.	2-2.5 c.	2-2.5 c.	2.5-3.5 c.	3.5-4.5 c.	3.5-4.5 c.
Vegetables	1.5-2 c.	2-2.5 c.	2.5-3 c.	2.5-3 c.	3-3.5 c.	3.5-4.5 c.	4.5-5 c.	4.5-5 c.
Grains	5 oz-eq.	5-6 oz-eq.	6-7 oz-eq.	6-7 oz-eq.	7-8 oz-eq.	8-9 oz-eq.	9-10 oz-eq.	10-11 oz-eq.
Meat & Beans	4 oz-eq.	5 oz-eq.	5-5.5 oz-eq.	5.5-6.5 oz-eq.	6.5-7 oz-eq.	7-7.5 oz-eq.	7-7.5 oz-eq.	7.5-8 oz-eq.
Milk	2-3 c.	3 c.	3 c.	3 c.	3 c.	3 c.	3 c.	3 c.
Healthy Oils	4 tsp.	5 tsp.	5 tsp.	6 tsp.	6 tsp.	7 tsp.	8 tsp.	8 tsp.

Day/Date:

Breakfast: _____

Lunch: _____

Dinner: _____

Snacks: _____

GROUP	FRUITS	VEGETABLES	GRAINS	MEAT & BEANS	MILK	OILS
Goal Amount						
Estimate Your Total						
Total Calories						

Physical Activity: _____ Spiritual Activity: _____

Steps/Miles/Minutes: _____ My Emotions Today: ❑ Happy   ❑ Sad   ❑ Stressed

Day/Date:

Breakfast: _____

Lunch: _____

Dinner: _____

Snacks: _____

GROUP	FRUITS	VEGETABLES	GRAINS	MEAT & BEANS	MILK	OILS
Goal Amount						
Estimate Your Total						
Total Calories						

Physical Activity: _____ Spiritual Activity: _____

Steps/Miles/Minutes: _____ My Emotions Today: ❑ Happy   ❑ Sad   ❑ Stressed

Day/Date:

Breakfast: _____

Lunch: _____

Dinner: _____

Snacks: _____

GROUP	FRUITS	VEGETABLES	GRAINS	MEAT & BEANS	MILK	OILS
Goal Amount						
Estimate Your Total						
Total Calories						

Physical Activity: _____ Spiritual Activity: _____

Steps/Miles/Minutes: _____ My Emotions Today: ❑ Happy   ❑ Sad   ❑ Stressed

Day/Date:

Breakfast: _____

Lunch: _____

Dinner: _____

Snacks: _____

GROUP	FRUITS	VEGETABLES	GRAINS	MEAT & BEANS	MILK	OILS
Goal Amount						
Estimate Your Total						
Total Calories						

Physical Activity: _____ Spiritual Activity: _____

Steps/Miles/Minutes: _____ My Emotions Today: ❏ Happy ❏ Sad ❏ Stressed

....

Day/Date:

Breakfast: _____

Lunch: _____

Dinner: _____

Snacks: _____

GROUP	FRUITS	VEGETABLES	GRAINS	MEAT & BEANS	MILK	OILS
Goal Amount						
Estimate Your Total						
Total Calories						

Physical Activity: _____ Spiritual Activity: _____

Steps/Miles/Minutes: _____ My Emotions Today: ❏ Happy ❏ Sad ❏ Stressed

....

Day/Date:

Breakfast: _____

Lunch: _____

Dinner: _____

Snacks: _____

GROUP	FRUITS	VEGETABLES	GRAINS	MEAT & BEANS	MILK	OILS
Goal Amount						
Estimate Your Total						
Total Calories						

Physical Activity: _____ Spiritual Activity: _____

Steps/Miles/Minutes: _____ My Emotions Today: ❏ Happy ❏ Sad ❏ Stressed

....

Day/Date:

Breakfast: _____

Lunch: _____

Dinner: _____

Snacks: _____

GROUP	FRUITS	VEGETABLES	GRAINS	MEAT & BEANS	MILK	OILS
Goal Amount						
Estimate Your Total						
Total Calories						

Physical Activity: _____ Spiritual Activity: _____

Steps/Miles/Minutes: _____ My Emotions Today: ❏ Happy ❏ Sad ❏ Stressed

....

Live It Tracker

Name: _____ Date: _____ Week #: _____

Loss/gain _____ lbs.   Calorie Range: _____   My food goal for the week: _____

Activity Level: None, < 30 min/day, 30-60 min/day, 60+ min/day   My activity goal for the week: _____

My spiritual goal for the week: _____

Group	Daily Calories							
	1300-1400	1500-1600	1700-1800	1900-2000	2100-2200	2300-2400	2500-2600	2700-2800
Fruits	1.5-2 c.	1.5-2 c.	1.5-2 c.	2-2.5 c.	2-2.5 c.	2.5-3.5 c.	3.5-4.5 c.	3.5-4.5 c.
Vegetables	1.5-2 c.	2-2.5 c.	2.5-3 c.	2.5-3 c.	3-3.5 c.	3.5-4.5 c.	4.5-5 c.	4.5-5 c.
Grains	5 oz-eq.	5-6 oz-eq.	6-7 oz-eq.	6-7 oz-eq.	7-8 oz-eq.	8-9 oz-eq.	9-10 oz-eq.	10-11 oz-eq.
Meat & Beans	4 oz-eq.	5 oz-eq.	5-5.5 oz-eq.	5.5-6.5 oz-eq.	6.5-7 oz-eq.	7-7.5 oz-eq.	7-7.5 oz-eq.	7.5-8 oz-eq.
Milk	2-3 c.	3 c.	3 c.	3 c.	3 c.	3 c.	3 c.	3 c.
Healthy Oils	4 tsp.	5 tsp.	5 tsp.	6 tsp.	6 tsp.	7 tsp.	8 tsp.	8 tsp.

Day/Date:

Breakfast: _____
Lunch: _____
Dinner: _____
Snacks: _____

GROUP	FRUITS	VEGETABLES	GRAINS	MEAT & BEANS	MILK	OILS
Goal Amount						
Estimate Your Total						
Total Calories						

Physical Activity: _____   Spiritual Activity: _____
Steps/Miles/Minutes: _____   My Emotions Today: ❑ Happy   ❑ Sad   ❑ Stressed

Day/Date:

Breakfast: _____
Lunch: _____
Dinner: _____
Snacks: _____

GROUP	FRUITS	VEGETABLES	GRAINS	MEAT & BEANS	MILK	OILS
Goal Amount						
Estimate Your Total						
Total Calories						

Physical Activity: _____   Spiritual Activity: _____
Steps/Miles/Minutes: _____   My Emotions Today: ❑ Happy   ❑ Sad   ❑ Stressed

Day/Date:

Breakfast: _____
Lunch: _____
Dinner: _____
Snacks: _____

GROUP	FRUITS	VEGETABLES	GRAINS	MEAT & BEANS	MILK	OILS
Goal Amount						
Estimate Your Total						
Total Calories						

Physical Activity: _____   Spiritual Activity: _____
Steps/Miles/Minutes: _____   My Emotions Today: ❑ Happy   ❑ Sad   ❑ Stressed

Day/Date:

Breakfast: _____
Lunch: _____
Dinner: _____
Snacks: _____

GROUP	FRUITS	VEGETABLES	GRAINS	MEAT & BEANS	MILK	OILS
Goal Amount						
Estimate Your Total						
Total Calories						

Physical Activity: _____　Spiritual Activity: _____
Steps/Miles/Minutes: _____　My Emotions Today: ❑ Happy　❑ Sad　❑ Stressed

---

Day/Date:

Breakfast: _____
Lunch: _____
Dinner: _____
Snacks: _____

GROUP	FRUITS	VEGETABLES	GRAINS	MEAT & BEANS	MILK	OILS
Goal Amount						
Estimate Your Total						
Total Calories						

Physical Activity: _____　Spiritual Activity: _____
Steps/Miles/Minutes: _____　My Emotions Today: ❑ Happy　❑ Sad　❑ Stressed

---

Day/Date:

Breakfast: _____
Lunch: _____
Dinner: _____
Snacks: _____

GROUP	FRUITS	VEGETABLES	GRAINS	MEAT & BEANS	MILK	OILS
Goal Amount						
Estimate Your Total						
Total Calories						

Physical Activity: _____　Spiritual Activity: _____
Steps/Miles/Minutes: _____　My Emotions Today: ❑ Happy　❑ Sad　❑ Stressed

---

Day/Date:

Breakfast: _____
Lunch: _____
Dinner: _____
Snacks: _____

GROUP	FRUITS	VEGETABLES	GRAINS	MEAT & BEANS	MILK	OILS
Goal Amount						
Estimate Your Total						
Total Calories						

Physical Activity: _____　Spiritual Activity: _____
Steps/Miles/Minutes: _____　My Emotions Today: ❑ Happy　❑ Sad　❑ Stressed

Live It Tracker

Name: _____ Date: _____ Week #: _____

Loss/gain _____ lbs.　Calorie Range: _____　My food goal for the week: _____

_____

Activity Level:　None,　< 30 min/day,　30-60 min/day,　60+ min/day　My activity goal for the week: _____

My spiritual goal for the week: _____

Group	Daily Calories							
	1300-1400	1500-1600	1700-1800	1900-2000	2100-2200	2300-2400	2500-2600	2700-2800
Fruits	1.5-2 c.	1.5-2 c.	1.5-2 c.	2-2.5 c.	2-2.5 c.	2.5-3.5 c.	3.5-4.5 c.	3.5-4.5 c.
Vegetables	1.5-2 c.	2-2.5 c.	2.5-3 c.	2.5-3 c.	3-3.5 c.	3.5-4.5 c.	4.5-5 c.	4.5-5 c.
Grains	5 oz-eq.	5-6 oz-eq.	6-7 oz-eq.	6-7 oz-eq.	7-8 oz-eq.	8-9 oz-eq.	9-10 oz-eq.	10-11 oz-eq.
Meat & Beans	4 oz-eq.	5 oz-eq.	5-5.5 oz-eq.	5.5-6.5 oz-eq.	6.5-7 oz-eq.	7-7.5 oz-eq.	7-7.5 oz-eq.	7.5-8 oz-eq.
Milk	2-3 c.	3 c.	3 c.	3 c.	3 c.	3 c.	3 c.	3 c.
Healthy Oils	4 tsp.	5 tsp.	5 tsp.	6 tsp.	6 tsp.	7 tsp.	8 tsp.	8 tsp.

Day/Date:

Breakfast: _____
Lunch: _____
Dinner: _____
Snacks: _____

GROUP	FRUITS	VEGETABLES	GRAINS	MEAT & BEANS	MILK	OILS
Goal Amount						
Estimate Your Total						
Total Calories						

Physical Activity: _____　Spiritual Activity: _____
Steps/Miles/Minutes: _____　My Emotions Today: ❏ Happy　❏ Sad　❏ Stressed

Day/Date:

Breakfast: _____
Lunch: _____
Dinner: _____
Snacks: _____

GROUP	FRUITS	VEGETABLES	GRAINS	MEAT & BEANS	MILK	OILS
Goal Amount						
Estimate Your Total						
Total Calories						

Physical Activity: _____　Spiritual Activity: _____
Steps/Miles/Minutes: _____　My Emotions Today: ❏ Happy　❏ Sad　❏ Stressed

Day/Date:

Breakfast: _____
Lunch: _____
Dinner: _____
Snacks: _____

GROUP	FRUITS	VEGETABLES	GRAINS	MEAT & BEANS	MILK	OILS
Goal Amount						
Estimate Your Total						
Total Calories						

Physical Activity: _____　Spiritual Activity: _____
Steps/Miles/Minutes: _____　My Emotions Today: ❏ Happy　❏ Sad　❏ Stressed

Day/Date: _____

Breakfast: _____

Lunch: _____

Dinner: _____

Snacks: _____

GROUP	FRUITS	VEGETABLES	GRAINS	MEAT & BEANS	MILK	OILS
Goal Amount						
Estimate Your Total						
Total Calories						

Physical Activity: _____ Spiritual Activity: _____

Steps/Miles/Minutes: _____ My Emotions Today: ❑ Happy ❑ Sad ❑ Stressed

---

Day/Date: _____

Breakfast: _____

Lunch: _____

Dinner: _____

Snacks: _____

GROUP	FRUITS	VEGETABLES	GRAINS	MEAT & BEANS	MILK	OILS
Goal Amount						
Estimate Your Total						
Total Calories						

Physical Activity: _____ Spiritual Activity: _____

Steps/Miles/Minutes: _____ My Emotions Today: ❑ Happy ❑ Sad ❑ Stressed

---

Day/Date: _____

Breakfast: _____

Lunch: _____

Dinner: _____

Snacks: _____

GROUP	FRUITS	VEGETABLES	GRAINS	MEAT & BEANS	MILK	OILS
Goal Amount						
Estimate Your Total						
Total Calories						

Physical Activity: _____ Spiritual Activity: _____

Steps/Miles/Minutes: _____ My Emotions Today: ❑ Happy ❑ Sad ❑ Stressed

---

Day/Date: _____

Breakfast: _____

Lunch: _____

Dinner: _____

Snacks: _____

GROUP	FRUITS	VEGETABLES	GRAINS	MEAT & BEANS	MILK	OILS
Goal Amount						
Estimate Your Total						
Total Calories						

Physical Activity: _____ Spiritual Activity: _____

Steps/Miles/Minutes: _____ My Emotions Today: ❑ Happy ❑ Sad ❑ Stressed

let's count our miles!

Join the 100-Mile Club this Session

Can't walk that mile yet? Don't be discouraged! There are exercises you can do to strengthen your body and burn those extra calories. Keep a record on your Live It Tracker of the number of minutes you do these common physical activities, convert those minutes to miles following the chart below, and then mark off each mile you have completed on the chart found on the back of the back cover. Report your miles to your 100-Mile Club representative when you first arrive each week. Remember, you are not competing with anyone else . . . just yourself. Your job is to strive to reach 100 miles before the last meeting in this session. You can do it—just keep on moving!

Walking

slowly, 2 MPH	30 min.	= 156 cal.	= 1 mile
moderately, 3 MPH	20 min.	= 156 cal.	= 1 mile
very briskly, 4 MPH	15 min.	= 156 cal.	= 1 mile
speed walking	10 min.	= 156 cal.	= 1 mile
up stairs	13 min.	= 159 cal.	= 1 mile

Running/Jogging

	10 min.	= 156 cal.	= 1 mile

Cycling Outdoors

slowly, <10 MPH	20 min.	= 156 cal.	= 1 mile
light effort, 10-12 MPH	12 min.	= 156 cal.	= 1 mile
moderate effort, 12-14 MPH	10 min.	= 156 cal.	= 1 mile
vigorous effort, 14-16 MPH	7.5 min.	= 156 cal.	= 1 mile
very fast, 16-19 MPH	6.5 min.	= 152 cal.	= 1 mile

Sports Activities

Playing tennis (singles)	10 min.	= 156 cal.	= 1 mile
Swimming			
light to moderate effort	11 min.	= 152 cal.	= 1 mile
fast, vigorous effort	7.5 min.	= 156 cal.	= 1 mile
Softball	15 min.	= 156 cal.	= 1 mile
Golf	20 min.	= 156 cal	= 1 mile
Rollerblading	6.5 min.	= 152 cal.	= 1 mile
Ice skating	11 min.	= 152 cal.	= 1 mile

Jumping rope	7.5 min.	= 156 cal.	= 1 mile
Basketball	12 min.	= 156 cal.	= 1 mile
Soccer (casual)	15 min.	= 159 cal.	= 1 mile

Around the House

Mowing grass	22 min.	= 156 cal.	= 1 mile
Mopping, sweeping, vacuuming	19.5 min.	= 155 cal.	= 1 mile
Cooking	40 min.	= 160 cal.	= 1 mile
Gardening	19 min.	= 156 cal.	= 1 mile
Housework (general)	35 min.	= 156 cal.	= 1 mile
Ironing	45 min.	= 153 cal.	= 1 mile
Raking leaves	25 min.	= 150 cal.	= 1 mile
Washing car	23 min.	= 156 cal.	= 1 mile
Washing dishes	45 min.	= 153 cal.	= 1 mile

At the Gym

Stair machine	8.5 min.	= 155 cal.	= 1 mile
Stationary bike			
slowly, 10 MPH	30 min.	= 156 cal.	= 1 mile
moderately, 10-13 MPH	15 min.	= 156 cal.	= 1 mile
vigorously, 13-16 MPH	7.5 min.	= 156 cal.	= 1 mile
briskly, 16-19 MPH	6.5 min.	= 156 cal.	= 1 mile
Elliptical trainer	12 min.	= 156 cal.	= 1 mile
Weight machines (used vigorously)	13 min.	= 152 cal.	= 1 mile
Aerobics			
low impact	15 min.	= 156 cal.	= 1 mile
high impact	12 min.	= 156 cal.	= 1 mile
water	20 min.	= 156 cal.	= 1 mile
Pilates	15 min.	= 156 cal.	= 1 mile
Raquetball (casual)	15 min.	= 159 cal.	= 1 mile
Stretching exercises	25 min.	= 150 cal.	= 1 mile
Weight lifting (also works for weight machines used moderately or gently)	30 min.	= 156 cal.	= 1 mile

Family Leisure

Playing piano	37 min.	= 155 cal.	= 1 mile
Jumping rope	10 min.	= 152 cal.	= 1 mile
Skating (moderate)	20 min.	= 152 cal.	= 1 mile
Swimming			
moderate	17 min.	= 156 cal.	= 1 mile
vigorous	10 min.	= 148 cal.	= 1 mile
Table tennis	25 min.	= 150 cal.	= 1 mile
Walk/run/play with kids	25 min.	= 150 cal.	= 1 mile

Week 2: Receive God's Blessing

*Now the Lord is the Spirit,
and where the Spirit of the
Lord is, there is freedom.*

Week 3: Step Out in Faith

*But you are a chosen people, a
royal priesthood, a holy nation,
a people belonging to God, that you
may declare the praises of him who
called you out of darkness
into his wonderful light.*

Start Losing
Start Living

Start Losing, Start Living
Scripture Memory Verses:

2 CORINTHIANS 3:17   HEBREWS 12:1
1 PETER 2:9   COLOSSIANS 3:16
COLOSSIANS 3:17   PSALM 9:10
GALATIANS 5:22-23   PHILIPPIANS 2:10-11
JAMES 4:7   ZEPHANIAH 3:17

How to Use These Cards:

Separate cards from the Bible study book. These cards are designed to be used when exercising. To do this, you may want to punch a hole in the upper left corner of the cards and place on a ring. When you have finished memorizing all the verses from one study, add the new Bible study cards to the ring and continue practicing the old verses while learning the new ones. Cards may be placed anywhere you will see them regularly—on the dashboard of your car, on a mirror, on a desk. After you have memorized the verse, begin using the reverse side of the card so the reference is connected to the verse. This is a great way to practice the verses you have already learned.

first place
4health

discover a new way to weight loss

2 CORINTHIANS 3:17

1 PETER 2:9

Week 6: Draw Nearer to God

Submit yourselves, then, to God. Resist the devil, and he will flee from you.

Week 7: Do Your Part in the Race

Therefore, since we are surrounded by such a great cloud of witnesses, let us throw off everything that hinders and the sin that so easily entangles, and let us run with perseverance the race marked out for us.

Week 4: Win Over Deception

And whatever you do, whether in word or deed, do it all in the name of the Lord Jesus, giving thanks to God the Father through him.

Week 5: Build a Legacy of Faithfulness

But the fruit of the Spirit is love, joy, peace, patience, kindness, goodness, faithfulness, gentleness and self-control. Against such things there is no law.

JAMES 4:7

COLOSSIANS 3:17

HEBREWS 12:1

GALATIANS 5:22-23